UNDERGROUND
CLINICAL VIGNETTES

· ·

NEUROLOGY

Classic Clinical Cases for
USMLE Step 2 Review [52 cases]

VIKAS BHUSHAN, MD
University of California, San Francisco, Class of 1991
Series Editor, Diagnostic Radiologist

TAO LE, MD
University of California, San Francisco, Class of 1996
Yale-New Haven Hospital, Resident in Internal Medicine

CHIRAG AMIN, MD
University of Miami, Class of 1996
Orlando Regional Medical Center, Resident in Orthopaedic Surgery

HOANG NGUYEN
Northwestern University, Class of 2000

NUTAN SHARMA, MD, PHD
Yale University School of Medicine, Resident in Neurology

©1999 by S2S Medical Publishing

NOTICE

The authors of this volume have taken care that the information contained herein is accurate and compatible with the standards generally accepted at the time of publication. Nevertheless, it is difficult to ensure that all the information given is entirely accurate for all circumstances. The publisher and authors do not guarantee the contents of this book and disclaim liability, loss, or damage incurred as a consequence, directly or indirectly, of the use and application of any of the contents of this volume.

DISTRIBUTED by Blackwell Science, Inc.
Editorial Office:
Commerce Place, 350 Main Street, Malden, Massachusetts 02148, USA

DISTRIBUTORS

USA

Commerce Place
350 Main Street
Malden, Massachusetts 02148
(Telephone orders: 800-215-1000 or
 781-388-8250;
 fax orders: 781-388-8270)

Canada

Login Brothers Book Company
324 Saulteaux Crescent
Winnipeg, Manitoba, R3J 3T2
(Telephone orders: 204-224-4068;
Telephone: 800-665-1148;
fax: 800-665-0103

Australia

Blackwell Science Pty Ltd.
54 University Street
Carlton, Victoria 3053
(Telephone orders: 03-9347-0300;
 fax orders: 03-9349-3016)

Outside North America and Australia

Blackwell Science, Ltd.
c/o Marston Book Service, Ltd.
P.O. Box 269
Abingdon
Oxon OX14 4YN
England
(Telephone orders: 44-01235-465500;
 fax orders: 44-01235-465555)

ISBN: 1-890061-26-3
TITLE: Underground Clinical Vignettes: Neurology

Editor: Andrea Fellows
Typesetter: Vikas Bhushan using MS Word97
Printed and bound by Capital City Press

Printed in the United States of America
99 00 01 02 6 5 4 3 2 1

Contributors

. . . .

KRIS ALDEN
University of Illinois, Chicago, MSTP

SUNIT DAS
Northwestern University, Class of 2000

JOSE M. FIERRO, MD
Brookdale Hospital, Resident in Medicine/Pediatrics

VISHAL PALL, MBBS
Government Medical College, Chandigarh, India, Class of 1996

VIPAL SONI
UCLA School of Medicine, Class of 1999

Faculty Reviewers

. . . .

RONALD COWAN, MD, PHD
McLean Hospital, Resident in Adult Psychiatry

MICHAEL MURPHY, MD, MPH
McLean Hospital, Resident in Adult Psychiatry

HUNED PATWA, MD
Yale University School of Medicine, Assistant Professor of Neurology

Acknowledgments

Throughout the production of this book, we have had the support of many friends and colleagues. Special thanks to our business manager, Gianni Le Nguyen. For expert computer support, Tarun Mathur and Alex Grimm. For additional copy editing services, Erica Simmons. For design suggestions, Sonia Santos and Elizabeth Sanders.

For authorship, editing, proofreading, and assistance across the vignette series, we collectively thank Chris Aiken, Kris Alden, Ted Amanios, Henry Aryan, Natalie Barteneva, MD, Adam Bennett, Ross Berkeley, MD, Archana Bindra, MBBS, Sanjay Bindra, MBBS, Aminah Bliss, Tamara Callahan, MD, MPP, Aaron Caughey, MD, MPP, Deanna Chin, Vladimir Coric, MD, Vladimir Coric, Sr., MD, Ronald Cowan, MD, PhD, Ryan Crowley, Daniel Cruz, Zubin Damania, Rama Dandamudi, MD, Sunit Das, Brian Doran, MD, Alea Eusebio, Thomas Farquhar, Jose Fierro, MBBS, Tony George, MD, Parul Goyal, Sundar Jayaraman, Eve Kaiyala, Sudhir Kakarla, Seth Karp, MD, Bertram Katzung, MD, PhD, Aaron Kesselheim, Jeff Knake, Sharon Kreijci, Christopher Kosgrove, MD, Warren Levinson, MD, PhD, Eric Ley, Joseph Lim, Andy Lin, Daniel Lee, Scott Lee, Samir Mehta, Gil Melmed, Michael Murphy, MD, MPH, Dan Neagu, MD, Deanna Nobleza, Craig Nodurft, Henry Nguyen, Linh Nguyen, MD, Vishal Pall, MBBS, Paul Pamphrus, MD, Thao Pham, MD, Michelle Pinto, Riva Rahl, Aashita Randeria, Rachan Reddy, Rajiv Roy, Diego Ruiz, Sanjay Sahgal, MD, Mustafa Saifee, MD, Louis Sanfillipo, MD, John Schilling, Sonal Shah, Nutan Sharma, MD, PhD, Andrew Shpall, Kristy Smith, Tanya Smith, Vipal Soni, Brad Spellberg, Merita Tan, MD, Eric Taylor, Jennifer Ty, Anne Vu, MD, Eunice Wang, MD, Lynna Wang, Andy Weiss, Thomas Yoo, and Ashraf Zaman, MBBS. Please let us know if your name has been missed or misspelled and we will be happy to make the change in the next edition.

For generously contributing images to the entire *Underground Clinical Vignette* Step 2 series, we collectively thank the staff at Blackwell Science in Oxford, Boston, and Berlin as well as:

- Alfred Cuschieri, Thomas P.J. Hennessy, Roger M. Greenhalgh, David I. Rowley, Pierce A. Grace (*Clinical Surgery*, © 1996 Blackwell Science), Figures 13.23, 13.35b, 13.51, 15.13, 15.2.

- John Axford (*Medicine*, © 1996 Blackwell Science), Figures f 3.10, 2.103a, 2.110b, 3.20a, 3.20b, 3.25b, 3.38a, 5.9Bi, 5.9Bii, 6.41a, 6.41b, 6.74b, 6.74c, 7.78ai, 7.78aii, 7.78b, 8.47b, 9.9e, f 3.17, f 3.36, f 3.37, f 5.27, f 5.28, f 5.45a, f 5.48, f 5.49a, f 5.50, f 5.65a, f 5.67, f 5.68, f 8.27a, AX10.120b, 11.63b, 11.63c, 11.68a, 11.68b, 11.68c, 12.37a, 12.37b.

Table of Contents

....

CASE	SUBSPECIALTY	NAME
1	Genetics	Friedreich's Ataxia
2	Genetics	Huntington's Disease
3	Genetics	von Hippel–Lindau Syndrome
4	ID	Aseptic Meningitis
5	ID	Bacterial Meningitis
6	ID	Creutzfeldt–Jakob Disease
7	ID	Herpes Encephalitis
8	ID	Neurosyphilis (Tabes Dorsalis)
9	ID	Polio
10	ID	Ramsay–Hunt Syndrome
11	ID	Subacute Sclerosing Panencephalitis
12	Neurology	Amyotrophic Lateral Sclerosis
13	Neurology	Bell's Palsy
14	Neurology	Brown–Séquard Syndrome
15	Neurology	Cerebral Palsy
16	Neurology	CVA - Broca's Aphasia
17	Neurology	CVA - Hypertensive
18	Neurology	CVA - Lacunar Stroke
19	Neurology	CVA - Left MCA Infarct
20	Neurology	CVA - Right MCA infarct
21	Neurology	CVA - Subarachnoid Hemorrhage
22	Neurology	CVA - Wernicke's Aphasia
23	Neurology	CVA due to Amyloid Angiopathy
24	Neurology	Dementia - Alzheimer's
25	Neurology	Dementia - Vascular
26	Neurology	Guillain–Barré Syndrome
27	Neurology	Horner's Syndrome
28	Neurology	Ménière's Disease
29	Neurology	Multiple Sclerosis
30	Neurology	Myasthenia Gravis
31	Neurology	Myotonic Dystrophy
32	Neurology	Normal Pressure Hydrocephalus
33	Neurology	Parkinson's Disease
34	Neurology	Peripheral Neuropathy due to Vincristine
35	Neurology	Pick's Disease
36	Neurology	Pseudotumor Cerebri
37	Neurology	Seizure - Absence
38	Neurology	Seizure - Complex Partial
39	Neurology	Seizure - Febrile

CASE	SUBSPECIALTY	NAME
40	Neurology	Seizure - Grand Mal
41	Neurology	Seizure - Metastatic Disease
42	Neurology	Spinal Cord Injury due to Trauma
43	Oncology	Astrocytoma
44	Oncology	Craniopharyngioma
45	Oncology	Glioblastoma Multiforme
46	Oncology	Medulloblastoma
47	Oncology	Neuroblastoma
48	Pain	Cluster Headache
49	Pain	Migraine Headache
50	Pain	Temporal Arteritis
51	Pain	Tension Headache
52	Pain	Trigeminal Neuralgia

Preface

This series was developed to address the nearly universal presence of clinical vignette questions on the USMLE Step 2. It is designed to supplement and complement *First Aid for the USMLE Step 2* (Appleton & Lange). Bidirectional cross-linking to appropriate High-Yield Facts in the second edition of *First Aid for the USMLE Step 2* has been implemented.

Each book uses a series of approximately 50 **"supra-prototypical" cases as a way to condense testable facts and associations.** The clinical vignettes in this series are designed to incorporate as many testable facts as possible into a cohesive and memorable clinical picture. The vignettes represent composites drawn from general and specialty textbooks, reference books, thousands of USMLE-style questions and the personal experience of the authors and reviewers. Additionally, we present "Associated Diseases" as a way to teach the most critical facts about a larger number of diseases that do not justify an entire case. **The "Associated Diseases" list is NOT complete and does not represent differential diagnoses.**

Although each case tends to present all the signs, symptoms, and diagnostic findings for a particular illness, **patients generally will not present with such a "complete" picture either clinically or on the Step 2 exam.** Cases are not meant to simulate a potential real patient or an exam vignette. All the **boldfaced "buzzwords" are for learning purposes** and are not necessarily expected to be found in any one patient with the disease. **Similarly, the images for each case are for learning purposes only, were derived from a variety of textbooks, and may not match the clinical vignette in all respects.** Images are labeled [A]–[D] and represent 1–4 images of varying sizes, with locations corresponding to a left-to-right, top-to-bottom lettering system.

Definitions of selected important terms are placed within the vignettes in (= SMALL CAPS) in parentheses. Other parenthetical remarks often refer to the pathophysiology or mechanism of disease. The format should also help students learn to present cases succinctly during oral "bullet" presentations on clinical rotations. The cases are meant to be read as a condensed review, not as a primary reference.

The information provided in this book has been prepared with a great deal of thought and careful research. This book should not, however, be considered your sole source of information. Corrections, suggestions, and submissions of new cases are encouraged and will be acknowledged and incorporated in future editions.

Abbreviations

ABCs - airway/breathing/circulation
ABGs - arterial blood gases
ADH - antidiuretic hormone
ANA - antinuclear antibody
ASO - anti-streptolysin O
AV - arteriovenous
BP - blood pressure
BUN - blood urea nitrogen
CAA - cerebral amyloid angiopathy
CAD - coronary artery disease
CBC - complete blood count
CJD - Creutzfeldt–Jakob disease
CK - creatine kinase
CN - cranial nerve
CNS - central nervous system
CSF - cerebrospinal fluid
CT - computed tomography
CVA - cerebrovascular accident
CXR - chest x-ray
DTRs - deep tendon reflexes
DVT - deep venous thrombosis
EBV - Epstein–Barr virus
ECG - electrocardiography
Echo - echocardiography
EEG - electroencephalography
ELISA - enzyme-linked immunosorbent assay
EMG - electromyography
ESR - erythrocyte sedimentation rate
FTA-ABS - fluorescent treponemal antibody absorption
GI - gastrointestinal
HIV - human immunodeficiency virus
HPI - history of present illness
HR - heart rate
HSV - herpes simplex virus
ICA - internal carotid artery
ICP - intracranial pressure
ID/CC - identification and chief complaint
IDDM - insulin-dependent diabetes mellitus
Ig - immunoglobulin
IM - intramuscular

Abbreviations - continued

INH - isoniazid
KUB - kidneys/ureter/bladder
LDL - low-density lipoprotein
LFTs - liver function tests
LMN - lower motor neuron
LP - lumbar puncture
LV - left ventricular
LVH - left ventricular hypertrophy
Lytes - electrolytes
MAO - monoamine oxidase
MCA - middle cerebral artery
MI - myocardial infarction
MPTP - 1-methyl-4-phenyl-1,2,3,6-tetrahydropyridine
MR - magnetic resonance (imaging)
MS - multiple sclerosis
NIDDM - non-insulin-dependent diabetes mellitus
NSAID - nonsteroidal anti-inflammatory drug
Nuc - nuclear medicine
PBS - peripheral blood smear
PE - physical exam
PFTs - pulmonary function tests
PMN - polymorphonuclear leukocyte
PT - prothrombin time
PTT - partial thromboplastin time
RPR - rapid plasma reagin
SAH - subarachnoid hemorrhage
SaO_2 - arterial blood oxygen saturation
SIADH - syndrome of inappropriate secretion of ADH
SSPE - subacute sclerosing panencephalitis
STD - sexually transmitted disease
TFTs - thyroid function tests
tPA - tissue plasminogen activator
TSH - thyroid-stimulating hormone
UA - urinalysis
UMN - upper motor neuron
URI - upper respiratory infection
US - ultrasound
UTI - urinary tract infection
VDRL - Venereal Disease Research Laboratory
VMA - vanillylmandelic acid
VS - vital signs
WBC - white blood cell

ID/CC	A **10-year-old** male is seen by a neurologist because of **progressive difficulty walking** and **diminution of vision.**
HPI	The patient has a **right foot deformity** (pes cavus). After suffering two episodes of syncope, he was diagnosed with **hypertrophic cardiomyopathy** by a cardiologist. His parents give a history of consanguineous marriage; **an uncle,** who had a similar illness, **died of cardiac complications.**
PE	VS: normal. PE: wide-based **ataxia;** nystagmus; dysarthria; **areflexia** in lower extremities; **Babinski's present; joint position sense** and vibration sense **lost in lower limbs;** pain and temperature sensations intact; intellect normal; 4/5 strength in lower extremities with 4+ strength in select muscle groups in upper extremities; curve in spine (scoliosis); optic atrophy.
Labs	Elevated blood glucose (200 mg/dL; indicative of overt **diabetes mellitus**).
Imaging	N/A
Pathogenesis	Friedreich's ataxia exhibits an **autosomal-recessive inheritance;** the gene locus has been mapped to chromosome 9. Classically, **three long tracts degenerate:** the pyramidal, dorsal, and spinocerebellar. Accompanying abnormalities include **cardiomyopathy,** skeletal abnormalities, optic atrophy, and an increased incidence of diabetes mellitus.
Epidemiology	Presents in children and involves ataxia with progressive involvement of all the extremities. The mean age of death is 31.
Management	No specific treatment is available.
Complications	**Cardiomyopathy is often the cause of death,** usually before age 40. Progressive neurologic decompensation results in loss of ambulation within five years after the onset of symptoms.
Associated Diseases	◼ Olivopontocerebellar Atrophy Also known as spinocerebellar ataxia; inherited as an autosomal-dominant trait; presents with adult-onset cerebellar ataxia, dysarthria, and extrapyramidal signs; there is no effective treatment.

1.   **FRIEDREICH'S ATAXIA**

◘ **Vitamin B12 Deficiency** Cofactor for DNA and myelin synthesis; deficiency is due to malabsorption (sprue, enteritis, *Diphyllobothrium latum* infection), absence of intrinsic factor (pernicious anemia), prolonged dietary deficiency (as in vegans), or terminal ileum disease; presents with anemia, degenerative changes in the spinal cord (especially the posterior columns and the corticospinal tracts), and peripheral neuropathies; hypersegmented PMNs, megaloblastic RBCs, and decreased serum vitamin B_{12}; treat the underlying disorder, IM vitamin B_{12}.

ID/CC	A **38-year-old** woman presents with a one-year history of progressive, **abrupt, involuntary jerking movements** of limbs (= CHOREA) with **diminished intellectual functioning.**
HPI	The patient's family first noted her inability to button clothes. Movements began with facial twitches and now are coarse, **purposeless, dancelike movements of the extremities** that disappear during sleep. Family members also complain that the patient is depressed, irritable, impulsive, and emotionally labile. For the past six months, she has displayed memory impairment. The patient's **mother died of "dementia"** at the age of 55, and her **brother was placed in a nursing home** at the age of 48.
PE	VS: normal. PE: blunted affect; unable to follow complex (three-step) commands; **lack of verbal and perceptual skills; deficits in attention,** organization, and sequencing abilities (due to frontal system dysfunction); short-term memory defective; diminished muscle tone.
Labs	**Trinucleotide repeat** in Huntington gene on chromosome 4p.
Imaging	**[A]** CT-Head: bilateral cerebral atrophy; rounding (due to caudate atrophy) and enlargement of the anterior horns of the lateral ventricles.
Pathogenesis	An **autosomal-dominant** condition with **100% penetrance** characterized by widespread loss of neurons in the neostriatum, it is a chronic, progressive neurodegenerative disorder. The function of the Huntington gene is unknown. Successive generations exhibit **lengthening of the trinucleotide repeat (=** GENETIC ANTICIPATION) and thus experience onset at progressively **younger ages.**
Epidemiology	Symptoms usually begin between 35 and 45 years.
Management	No treatment is available for the underlying neurologic disease. **Haloperidol,** perphenazine, or drugs that **block dopamine receptors** or **deplete brain monoamines** reduce choreiform movements. Tricyclic antidepressants or SSRIs for depression. Concurrent use of MAO inhibitors and tricyclic antidepressants is

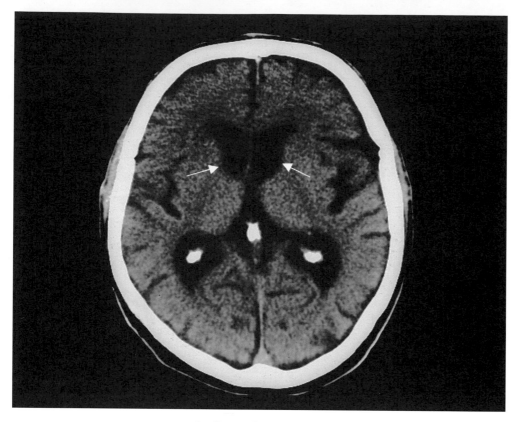

contraindicated.

Complications   Patients may develop dysphagia and become progressively rigid and bedridden. Death is typically due to infection (pneumonia, UTI).

Associated Diseases   ◻ **Rheumatic Fever** Complication of group A streptococcal infection, secondary to autoantibodies directed against joints and heart valves; presents > 1 week after throat infection with migratory polyarthritis, endocarditis, and rash; antistreptococcal antibodies (e.g., ASO); treat with aspirin and penicillin; complications include permanent valvular disease.

◻ **Tardive Dyskinesia** Late-occurring abnormal choreoathetoid movements associated with antipsychotics (dopamine antagonists); presents with abnormal facial gestures and lip smacking; treat by discontinuing the offending agent; the disorder is typically irreversible.

HUNTINGTON'S DISEASE

ID/CC	A 31-year-old female presents with **headaches, nausea, and vomiting** of two months' duration.
HPI	The headaches have slowly increased in severity over the past month. She denies any change in vision or motor weakness. Her **mother died of cancer** at the age of 28.
PE	VS: normal. PE: speech appropriate; mild papilledema in right disk; left disk not well visualized owing to **enlarged globular blood vessel** (= HAMARTOMA); finger-to-nose exam significant for mild **dysmetria**; gait slightly **wide-based;** tandem gait severely impaired; sensory exam intact.
Labs	CBC: **polycythemia** (due to ectopic erythropoietin production by hemangioblastoma).
Imaging	CT-Brain: large, low-density, **cystic-appearing mass** in the midline of the **cerebellum.** CT-Abdomen: multiple **bilateral renal cysts.**
Pathogenesis	Von Hippel–Lindau disease is characterized by cerebellar **hemangioblastomas** or **retinal angiomas** and by the presence of **cysts in at least one visceral organ.** Within the same family, all gradations of the syndrome may be found. The gene locus for von Hippel–Lindau syndrome has been mapped to **chromosome 3p.**
Epidemiology	Becomes symptomatic during adult life and has an **autosomal-dominant** pattern of inheritance.
Management	**Surgical excision** of hemangioblastomas (surgical approach aided by cerebral angiogram). Annual ophthalmologic exams to screen for **retinal hemangioblastoma.**
Complications	Retinal hemangioblastoma, recurrence of hemangioblastoma, adrenal abnormalities (pheochromocytoma, adrenal medulla cyst, adrenal cortical hyperplasia), and renal carcinoma.
Associated Diseases	◻ **AV Malformation** Congenital vascular malformations, more common in men; CNS AVMs present with headache and seizures; contrast CT, angiography, and MR reveal the AVM; treat with coiling, surgical excision or embolization; complications include rupture causing intracerebral or subarachnoid hemorrhage.

ID/CC	A 25-year-old woman presents with **headache,** fever, and **neck stiffness** of two days' duration.
HPI	She had a URI two weeks ago. She now also complains of nausea and **vomiting.**
PE	VS: fever. PE: alert and oriented; **mild nuchal rigidity; Kernig's and Brudzinski's negative;** no focal deficits; funduscopy normal.
Labs	CBC: normal. Lytes: normal (serum glucose 125 mg/dL). LP: opening pressure 11 cm water; clear; CSF **glucose 100 mg/dL; 20 WBCs with 90% lymphocytes; mildly raised protein;** CSF Gram stain reveals no organisms.
Imaging	CT-Head: normal.
Pathogenesis	Meningitis is an inflammation of the leptomeninges and presents as CSF pleocytosis. Enteroviruses, mumps virus, arborvirus, HSV, HIV, and medications (ibuprofen) are causes of aseptic meningitis.
Epidemiology	Incidence is 1 in 10,000 per year. A specific pathogen is rarely identified.
Management	Treat with bed rest, analgesics, and antipyretics. Typically runs a benign, short (two- to three-day) course.
Complications	The prognosis is excellent in adults; rare complications in infants include hearing loss and learning disabilities.

FIRST AID 2 p. 202

Associated Diseases

◘ **Bacterial Meningitis** Infection of the meninges, most commonly by *Streptococcus pneumoniae* in adults; presents with fever, neck stiffness, positive Kernig's sign, altered mental status, and seizures; CSF reveals organisms on Gram stain, high protein, low glucose, and many neutrophils; treat empirically with ceftriaxone until CSF cultures return; complications include cranial nerve palsies and hydrocephalus.

◘ **Meningococcemia** Systemically disseminated infection with *Neisseria meningitidis;* more commonly seen in those with terminal complement component (C5–C8) deficiency; presents with sudden fever, chills, severe headache, meningeal signs, and petechial rash; hypoglycemia, hyperkalemia, and hyponatremia; gram-negative diplococci in blood, possibly in CSF; gross

ASEPTIC MENINGITIS

pathology reveals bilateral adrenal hemorrhage; treat
with penicillin G, rifampin for close contacts;
complications include fulminant adrenal infarction; also
called Waterhouse–Friderichsen syndrome.

ASEPTIC MENINGITIS

ID/CC	A 50-year-old male presents with **high fever** with chills, severe **headache,** and a **declining mental status.**
HPI	The patient is homeless and had been complaining of cough and fever for the last week. He was found in a stupor.
PE	VS: fever (39.5 C); **tachycardia** (HR 130); tachypnea; hypotension (BP 90/60). PE: nonverbal, confused, disoriented, and unable to follow commands; no skin rashes (meningococcal meningitis less likely); nuchal rigidity; **Kernig's and Brudzinski's positive;** no cranial nerve palsies; Babinski's absent; funduscopy normal.
Labs	CBC: leukocytosis (20,000). Normal serum glucose (110 mg/dL). LP: **opening pressure 25 cm water; 2,000 WBCs/uL (90% PMNs); glucose 20 mg/dL; protein 170 mg/dL;** CSF Gram stain reveals **gram-positive cocci** in chains. Culture yields *S. pneumoniae*.
Imaging	CT-Head: normal.
Pathogenesis	Bacteria may infiltrate the meninges via the blood or from adjacent structures; **hematogenous spread is most common** and typically occurs via the upper respiratory tract. Low glucose in the CSF, high protein, and marked pleocytosis are characteristic of bacterial meningitis; **Gram stain,** which is positive in 80% of cases, is diagnostic. The most common organisms involved are *H. influenzae, Neisseria meningitidis,* and *S. pneumoniae.*
Epidemiology	*S. pneumoniae* **is the most common cause of meningitis in adults** and the second most common cause in children > 6 years of age.
Management	Empiric IV ceftriaxone; then narrow the antibiotic spectrum when the organism is isolated. In cases of increased ICP, **steroids** should be used.
Complications	Pneumococcal meningitis has a significant mortality rate and is associated with residual neurologic deficits, seizures, and sepsis. Coma and pneumonia are associated with a poor prognosis. **FIRST AID 2** p. 202
Associated Diseases	N/A

BACTERIAL MENINGITIS

ID/CC	A **60-year-old** male presents with a rapidly progressive **change in mental status** over the past two months with an **inability to concentrate** and **memory impairment.**
HPI	His relatives have noticed increased somnolence, changes in his personality, and **twitching movements of the hands** and **difficulty walking** (due to ataxia) for several months.
PE	VS: normal. PE: no papilledema; normal speech; **ataxic gait** with **choreoathetotic movements** and **myoclonus;** normal DTRs; normal sensation; cranial nerves intact.
Labs	CBC/Lytes: normal. TFTs normal. LFTs: normal. LP: CSF analysis normal. EEG: **diffuse, slow background with superimposed sharp triphasic synchronous discharge complexes.**
Imaging	CT/MR-Brain: generalized cortical atrophy.
Pathogenesis	A **subacute encephalopathy of the spongiform type** that is caused by a slow-virus-like agent (= PRION) with a very long incubation period. Creutzfeldt–Jakob disease (CJD) gives rise to progressive dementia and associated myoclonus and may be **transmitted** by **corneal transplants, dura mater allografts,** contaminated **cadaveric growth hormone, EEG electrodes,** and **neurosurgical contamination.** Pathologic findings include softening of CNS tissue with vacuolization and secondary amyloidosis but no inflammatory reaction. Unlike Alzheimer's, there is very little cerebral atrophy owing to the rapid progression of the disease. CJD is diagnosed by brain biopsy after other causes of dementia have been ruled out.
Epidemiology	Occurs with greater frequency in the sixth decade of life; shows no gender predominance. Has a higher incidence within families and in certain geographical areas, such as Czechoslovakia, North Africa, and Chile. Closely associated with **kuru from New Guinea,** which is now a rare disease (was transmitted by some tribal traditions of eating human brains). The disease **progresses rapidly;** one-year survival is rare.
Management	**No specific treatment is available,** and the disease has a very **poor short-term prognosis.**

Complications	Coma and death.
Associated Diseases	◨ **Gerstmann–Sträussler–Scheinker syndrome** Rare spinocerebellar degeneration; hereditary; onset in mid-adulthood; presents with progressive ataxia, nystagmus, and extrapyramidal signs; there is no proven treatment.

◨ **Huntington's Disease** An autosomal-dominant disorder of movement and cognition; onset is during the 30s to 50s; presents with severe, progressive chorea and dementia; CT shows caudate degeneration; treat chorea with dopamine blockade (e.g., haloperidol); invariably fatal.

◨ **Syphilis** An STD caused by *Treponema pallidum* infection; divided into primary, secondary, tertiary, and congenital; primary presents with a painless chancre in the genital area; secondary presents with a diffuse maculopapular rash, especially on the palms and soles, and with condylomata lata; tertiary presents with aortic aneurysms, gumma formation, and neurologic disease; congenital presents with fetal death or congenital abnormalities; screen with VDRL or RPR; more specific tests are FTA-ABS and darkfield microscopy; treat with penicillin.

CREUTZFELDT–JAKOB DISEASE

ID/CC	A 30-year-old male complains of moderate **headache,** nausea, **vomiting, fever** with chills, and muscle aches for the past two days.
HPI	Three days ago, the patient's wife noted that he **started to "forget things."** He has also been unable to name familiar objects such as a radio. His wife has noted **speech difficulty** and episodes of irritable behavior over the past 24 hours. He has also been **smelling nonexistent odors** (olfactory hallucinations are common in HSV encephalitis).
PE	VS: fever (38.4 C); **tachycardia** (HR 120); **tachypnea** (RR 24). PE: mildly confused and disoriented; **mild nuchal rigidity;** speech notable for **paraphasic errors** (e.g., "shoon" instead of "spoon"); patient follows simple (one-step) commands and approximately 50% of complex (three-step) commands; he can draw a clock and bisect lines correctly (tests of nondominant parietal lobe function) and can add and subtract two-digit numbers but cannot perform simple (one-digit) multiplication problems; cranial nerves intact; motor strength 5/5 bilaterally; DTRs 2+ and symmetric throughout; patient withdraws limbs to painful stimuli.
Labs	CBC/Lytes: normal. PT/PTT, BUN, and creatinine normal. LFTs: normal. LP: opening pressure of 100 mm water; **protein elevated** (100 mg/dL); **glucose normal;** elevated WBC count with **mononuclear pleocytosis; red cells present;** CSF culture negative (positive in HSV-2).
Imaging	**[A]** and **[B]** CT-Brain: bilateral temporal lobe hypodensity (1). MR-Brain: **T2 hyperintensity** involving the cortex and white matter in the **temporal lobes.**
Pathogenesis	Ninety-five percent of cases are due to **HSV type 1.** The ports of entry are the oropharyngeal mucosa, conjunctiva, or broken skin; the virus **replicates locally and enters the sensory nerves.** From the sensory nerves, the virus is transported to the sensory nerve ganglia, where it remains latent. The factors that induce activation of the latent virus and the mechanism by which the virus targets the temporal lobes are not well understood.
Epidemiology	HSV encephalitis is the most common identified cause of acute sporadic viral encephalitis. HSV-1 encephalitis

HERPES ENCEPHALITIS

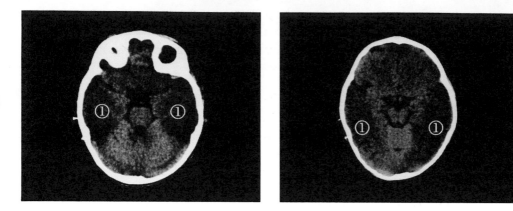

occurs in all age groups, in both sexes, and during all seasons.

Management   Untreated patients rapidly deteriorate to coma and death in 70% of cases. Treat with **IV acyclovir.** Mannitol and corticosteroids are given to relieve cerebral edema, and phenytoin is used to treat seizures. Repeat lumbar puncture after treatment to ensure that there is no residual infection.

Complications   Complications include persistent seizures and neurologic deficits. Amnesia is a prominent residual symptom.

Associated Diseases   ◻ **Bacterial Meningitis** Infection of the meninges, most commonly by *Streptococcus pneumoniae* in adults; presents with fever, neck stiffness, positive Kernig's sign, altered mental status, and seizures; CSF reveals organisms on Gram stain, high protein, low glucose, and many neutrophils; treat empirically with ceftriaxone until CSF cultures return; complications include cranial nerve palsies and hydrocephalus.

ID/CC	A 45-year-old male with a history of **untreated venereal disease** complains of **pain in his legs** and **difficulty walking,** especially in the dark.
HPI	For the past year, the patient has noted sporadic episodes of electric-like **"lightning" pain in his legs** that last for hours or days. He also complains of persistent numbness and tingling (feeling of "pins and needles") in his feet and has been **"stumbling"** whenever he turns quickly.
PE	VS: normal. PE: **discrepancy in pupillary size** (= ANISOCORIA); involved pupil **reacts poorly to light but normally to accommodation** (= ARGYLL– ROBERTSON PUPIL); cranial nerves grossly intact; motor exam 5/5 bilaterally throughout; DTRs 2+ and symmetric in upper extremities but **absent at patella and Achilles;** Babinski's absent bilaterally; sensory exam reveals **decreased vibratory and proprioception sense** in feet; **Romberg's sign positive;** patient maintains knees in an extended position; finger-to-nose intact bilaterally (tests cerebellar function).
Labs	CBC/Lytes: normal. PT/PTT and glucose normal; **serum FTA-ABS positive.** LP: **lymphocytic pleocytosis;** protein of 80 mg/dL; normal glucose; **positive FTA-ABS; positive oligoclonal bands** (FTA-ABS test is more sensitive and specific for the detection of treponemal antigens than VDRL).
Imaging	N/A
Pathogenesis	Tabes dorsalis is a form of **neurosyphilis** that is characterized by **chronic progressive demyelination** of the posterior column of the spinal cord, posterior sensory ganglia (dorsal root ganglia), and nerve roots. *Treponema pallidum,* a spirochete, is the causative organism; it usually invades the CNS 3–18 months after systemic infection occurs.
Epidemiology	The incidence of latent syphilis is 7.4 per 100,000 in the U.S.
Management	Treat with **IV penicillin.** If the patient is allergic to penicillin, he should undergo desensitization and then proceed with penicillin. Follow response to therapy by checking LP repeatedly over two years. Expect normalization of CSF VDRL by one year; relapse after

NEUROSYPHILIS (TABES DORSALIS)

two years of negative CSF is uncommon.

Complications   Complications include **Charcot's joints** (joint damage due to decreased sensation of lower limbs), incontinence secondary to neurogenic bladder, painless ulcers over pressure points, hearing loss, and visual loss due to uveitis, chorioretinitis, or optic neuritis. **Tabes crises** consist of abdominal pain and bladder dysfunction.

Associated Diseases   ◘ **Syphilis** An STD caused by *Treponema pallidum* infection; divided into primary, secondary, tertiary, and congenital; primary presents with a painless chancre in the genital area; secondary presents with a diffuse maculopapular rash, especially on the palms and soles, and with condylomata lata; tertiary presents with aortic aneurysms, gumma formation, and neurologic disease; congenital presents with fetal death or congenital abnormalities; screen with VDRL or RPR; more specific tests are FTA-ABS and darkfield microscopy; treat with penicillin.

ID/CC	A 15-year-old Amish male presents with a three-day history of progressive **leg weakness.**
HPI	The patient has **not had any immunizations.** His weakness has progressed such that he is now unable to climb stairs. He also complains of tingling in the legs but denies any weakness in his arms or any prior trauma.
PE	VS: fever (38.3 C); normal BP. PE: alert and oriented; CN II–XII intact; **motor tone** normal in both arms but **flaccid in both legs; motor strength 3/5 in both legs; DTRs absent bilaterally in patella and Achilles; sensory exam intact** to all primary modalities; sphincter tone normal.
Labs	CBC/LP: normal.
Imaging	N/A
Pathogenesis	The causative agent is **poliovirus** serotypes 1, 2, and 3. The virus **enters the body via the GI tract** and multiplies in the lymphoid tissue of the GI tract; it then spreads to the CNS via the bloodstream, where it attacks the **motor neurons of the spinal cord** and **brainstem.** Person-to-person spread is via the oral-oral or oral-fecal route.
Epidemiology	Because of effective mass immunization, the annual incidence of polio in the U.S. has markedly decreased. Outbreaks occur in unimmunized individuals and in those exposed to wild-type polio virus type I.
Management	There is no specific treatment. Airway maintenance and ventilatory support should be instituted as necessary. Prevention with immunization is essential.
Complications	**Autonomic instability** resulting in cardiac arrhythmias and wide variation in blood pressure. Bulbar polio may jeopardize respiratory center function.
Associated Diseases	◘ **Lyme Disease** Caused by the spirochete *Borrelia burgdorferi;* the vector is the *Ixodes* tick; presents with a migrating, target-shaped, erythematous rash called erythema migrans as well as with lymphadenopathy and arthritis; positive IgM ELISA for *B. burgdorferi;* treat with doxycycline.

ID/CC	A 50-year-old female presents with sudden-onset left-sided **facial weakness, hearing loss,** and **ear pain** of two days' duration.
HPI	The patient also has left-sided **throat pain** and **altered taste sensation.** She recently underwent radiation treatment for an unidentified lymphoma (immune-compromised state).
PE	**Vesicular rash** on left external ear (herpes zoster); **sensorineural hearing loss** on left side; taste absent on left anterior third of tongue; **left-sided peripheral facial palsy.**
Labs	CBC: lymphocytosis. LP: **elevated protein** in CSF. **Tzanck smear of vesicles positive.**
Imaging	CT-Head: no intracranial lesions or hemorrhage.
Pathogenesis	Herpes zoster reactivation is promoted by radiation and immune compromise, including that associated with lymphoproliferative disorders, HIV, and cytotoxic chemotherapy. The virus remains dormant in nerve roots and ganglia. Herpes zoster reactivation is also called **shingles;** when it involves the **seventh and eighth cranial nerves,** it is designated Ramsay–Hunt syndrome. The diagnosis of Ramsay–Hunt syndrome can generally be made on the basis of history and physical exam.
Epidemiology	The incidence in children is low; in adults, it is approximately 2.5 per 1,000 per year.
Management	**Acyclovir** has been shown to reduce the duration of the vesicular rash and diminish the likelihood of postherpetic neuralgia. **Corticosteroids** may also be used as adjuvant therapy to shorten the duration and reduce the chance of postherpetic neuralgia.
Complications	Hearing loss, reactivation of virus, meningoencephalitis in immune-compromised patients.
Associated Diseases	◻ **Bell's Palsy** The most common form of facial paralysis; idiopathic; rapid onset of usually unilateral facial weakness; treat with eye protection; a short corticosteroid course may speed recovery.

ID/CC	An **8-year-old boy** presents with **"jerking"** movements.
HPI	The boy has no significant medical history and does not have a regular pediatrician. His mother cannot remember if his vaccinations are up to date. He had **measles at 10 months of age** but has developed normally. In the last month, his grades at school have worsened considerably. Two days ago, his mother noted the onset of continuous "jerking" movements.
PE	VS: normal. PE: **lethargic** but able to cooperate; neck supple; cranial nerves intact; motor tone exceptional given continuous **myoclonic movements** involving all four extremities; DTRs 2+ and symmetric throughout; finger-to-nose exam reveals mild **dysmetria;** gait normal; sensation intact to pinprick in all four extremities.
Labs	CBC: normal. EEG: **burst suppression.** LP: normal opening pressure; normal protein and glucose with no white cells; CSF antibody titer **elevated** for **measles-specific antibodies.** No organisms on Gram stain; **elevated oligoclonal bands.**
Imaging	CT-Brain: cerebral edema and diffuse hypodense signal in white matter bilaterally.
Pathogenesis	Due to **accumulation of defective measles virus in neurons.** In those with subacute sclerosing panencephalitis (SSPE), neurons contain viral nucleic acid and proteins that cannot be integrated into viral particles. SSPE is characterized by **three clinical stages:** stage I is marked by behavioral and cognitive decline, stage II by motor dysfunction (spasticity, weakness) and often myoclonic jerks and seizures, and stage III by stupor, coma, and autonomic failure (loss of thermoregulation). Death occurs 1–3 years after onset of symptoms.
Epidemiology	Fewer than 10 cases per year in the U.S. Average age of onset is 6–8 years; the median interval between acute measles infection and SSPE is eight years. **Males** are affected three times more often than females. Large-scale measles vaccination programs have resulted in a 20-fold decrease in the risk of SSPE.
Management	**Supportive care;** antiepileptic treatment if seizures

11. **SUBACUTE SCLEROSING PANENCEPHALITIS**

occur.

Complications	Seizures, autonomic failure, coma, and death.
Associated Diseases	N/A

SUBACUTE SCLEROSING PANENCEPHALITIS

ID/CC	A **45-year-old male** complains of slowly **progressive muscle weakness** involving the **hands and lower limbs.**
HPI	He has had muscle wasting, weakness, rigidity, and slowness. He denies any incontinence or changes in his bowel habits. He has also noted difficulty walking (impaired gait).
PE	VS: normal. PE: **muscle atrophy,** weakness, wasting, **fasciculations,** loss of stretch reflexes, and bradykinesia noted in **upper extremities** bilaterally (LMN signs); **muscle rigidity, spasticity,** clonus, and hyperactive DTRs noted in bilateral **lower extremities** (UMN signs); **Babinski's present** (UMN sign); spastic gait; no sensory deficit.
Labs	Muscle biopsy shows **grouping of muscle fiber types** (as nerves die, adjacent nerves send buds to reinnervate muscle and fibers switch types). LP: mildly elevated protein (50 mg/dL) in CSF. EMG: **fasciculations** and evidence of **denervation** in upper extremities with **normal nerve conduction velocities.**
Imaging	CT/MR-Brain and Spinal Cord: normal.
Pathogenesis	Also known as **Lou Gehrig's disease.** The cause is unknown; it is usually sporadic and associated with an infectious etiology. Affects both **anterior horn cells** in the spinal cord and **UMNs** in the corticospinal tract, resulting in both UMN and LMN deficits. UMN and LMN signs may be asymmetric.
Epidemiology	**Males** are more likely to be affected than females. **Incidence rises after age 40** and continues to increase until about 80.
Management	**No specific treatment.** Symptomatic management is indicated, including anticholinergics to prevent drooling and braces and physical therapy to assist mobility and prevent contractures.
Complications	Dysphagia, respiratory compromise, and aspiration; **death within five years of symptom onset.**
Associated Diseases	N/A

AMYOTROPHIC LATERAL SCLEROSIS

ID/CC	A 45-year-old female presents with new-onset right-sided **facial weakness** and **drooping of the right side of the mouth.**
HPI	She complains of a sore right eye (due to drying of the cornea). She also becomes irritated upon hearing even minor noises, complaining that they are "too loud" (= HYPERACUSIS).
PE	Alert and oriented × 3; funduscopy normal; right-sided **paralysis of upper and lower face** such that eye cannot be closed tightly (or can easily be opened by physician); eyeball turns up on attempted closure (= BELL'S PHENOMENON); patient is **unable to raise right eyebrow** (= LOWER MOTOR NEURON RIGHT FACIAL PALSY); corner of mouth droops and **nasolabial fold** is **decreased;** voluntary and involuntary movements of mouth are paralyzed on right side (lips are drawn to opposite side); examination of right ear normal (to rule out herpetic Ramsay–Hunt syndrome); no other cranial nerve palsy found; no other neurologic deficit.
Labs	N/A
Imaging	CT-Head: no intracranial lesions or hemorrhage.
Pathogenesis	Bell's palsy is by definition **idiopathic.** Approximately 80% recover fully.
Epidemiology	The **most common form of facial paralysis.**
Management	**No specific treatment.** Artificial tears and taping the eye shut at night. High-dose corticosteroids may shorten the disease course.
Complications	Chronic paralysis in a minority of cases.
Associated Diseases	◻ **Cerebellopontine Angle Compression** An acoustic neuroma, meningioma, metastatic lesion, or cholesteatoma compressing the cerebellopontine angle; presents with unilateral hearing loss, tinnitus, vertigo, and facial nerve palsy; CT or MR demonstrates mass lesion; treat with radiation therapy to shrink the tumor or surgical resection; complications include increased ICP.

◻ **Lyme Disease** Caused by the spirochete *Borrelia burgdorferi;* the vector is the *Ixodes* tick; presents with a |

migrating, target-shaped, erythematous rash called erythema migrans as well as with lymphadenopathy and arthritis; positive IgM ELISA for *B. burgdorferi;* treat with doxycycline.

◘ **Mononeuritis Multiplex** A broad term describing a pattern of nerve dysfunction in which affected nerves are individually identifiable; common causes include polyarteritis nodosa, diabetes mellitus, rheumatoid arthritis, amyloidosis, HIV infection, and leprosy; presents with diffuse involvement of both motor and sensory peripheral nerves; nerve conduction studies demonstrate axonal damage; treat underlying disease.

◘ **Ramsay–Hunt Syndrome** Varicella-zoster virus reactivation in the geniculate ganglion of the facial nerve; presents with painful vesicles in the auditory canal and face and with facial palsy; Tzanck smear of lesions shows multinucleated giant cells; treat with intravenous acyclovir to shorten the outbreak.

ID/CC	A 17-year-old male who was **stabbed in the back** presents with **inability to use his left leg** along with stiffness and **loss of pain sensation in the right leg.**
HPI	The stab wound extended to the spinal cord at the level of L1 slightly to the left of the spinous process. Since the injury, the patient has been unable to move his left leg. He also complains of episodes of "tingling" of the distal left leg.
PE	VS: normal. PE: cranial nerves intact; motor exam demonstrates 5/5 strength bilaterally in upper extremities, 5/5 strength in right lower extremity, and 0/5 strength in left lower extremity; increased tone in left leg; DTRs 2+ and symmetric in upper extremities, 3+ in left patella and Achilles, and 2+ in right patella and Achilles; **diminished proprioception and vibration sense** in left leg; **loss of pain and temperature** sense in right leg; Babinski's present in left leg.
Labs	N/A
Imaging	MR-Spine: no intramedullary mass identified.
Pathogenesis	Due to **hemisection of the spinal cord.** This results in ipsilateral UMN signs below the lesion (hyperreflexia, spastic paralysis resulting from lateral corticospinal tract interruption), ipsilateral loss of vibration and proprioception sense (due to damage to the dorsal column), and contralateral loss of pain and temperature sensation (due to damage of the spinothalamic tract that decussated below lesion).
Epidemiology	Typically occurs secondary to **trauma** (e.g., bullet or stab wounds), spinal cord **tumor,** or fracture-dislocation causing compression.
Management	**Symptomatic relief** of hyperesthesias; phenytoin and carbamazepine are effective.
Complications	Limited mobility may result in pressure ulcers or URIs; the neurologic syndrome itself does not progress.
Associated Diseases	◘ **Cauda Equina Syndrome** A lesion affecting the nerve roots that branch off the end of the spinal cord (= CAUDA EQUINA); caused by disk herniation, tumor, paraspinal abscess, or hematoma; presents with low back pain, lower extremity sensory loss with sacral sparing,

BROWN-SÉQUARD SYNDROME

weakness, urinary and bowel incontinence, impotence, and loss of reflexes; CT or MR demonstrates the lesion; treatment is surgical decompression for disk herniation, radiotherapy and surgery for tumor, and antibiotics and incision and drainage for abscess.

◘ **Lumbar Spinal Stenosis** May mimic cord compression; usually due to congenital narrowing of the spinal canal exacerbated by degenerative osteoarthritic changes or hypertrophy of the facet joints, causing pressure on nerve roots; presents with pseudoclaudication (pain in the leg or back occurring during walking) relieved by sitting forward; CT/MR demonstrate spinal canal narrowing; treat with surgical decompression (laminectomy).

ID/CC	A 4-year-old female who was **born prematurely** presents with **difficulty walking.**
HPI	The child was born at 28 weeks. She reached all developmental milestones at the appropriate age with the exception of ambulation but has learned to walk within the past year. Her parents have noted that her **gait is clumsy and stiff** (= SPASTIC GAIT). She also has abnormal, **abrupt, jerky movements of her limbs** (= CHOREA) and sometimes **slow, writhing, continuous movements** (= ATHETOSIS).
PE	Motor strength 4/5 in both lower extremities and 5/5 in both upper extremities; **motor tone increased** in lower extremities but normal in upper extremities; DTRs 3+ bilaterally in lower extremities and 2+ bilaterally in upper extremities; **Moro's and asymmetrical tonic neck reflexes persist.**
Labs	N/A
Imaging	MR-Brain: **periventricular white matter disease.**
Pathogenesis	Cerebral palsy is a motor deficit of **unknown etiology** due to a nonprogressive lesion in the immature brain. The pathology may occur at any stage of brain development. Premature newborns may suffer from periventricular hemorrhage affecting the white matter, which primarily carries that portion of the corticospinal tract which is responsible for leg movement.
Epidemiology	Cerebral palsy is associated with **cerebral anoxia** at birth, **prematurity, trauma, embryologic malformations,** and **infection.**
Management	**Physical and occupational therapy** should be initiated at birth. Orthotic devices should be used if ambulation is significantly affected. Treat associated problems such as seizures and learning disabilities.
Complications	Complications depend on the severity of cerebral palsy. If mobility is severely limited, patients may suffer from pneumonia, UTIs, and decubitus ulcers. Associated problems include epilepsy, mental retardation, behavioral problems, and learning disabilities.
Associated Diseases	N/A

....

CEREBRAL PALSY

ID/CC	A 62-year-old right-handed male with a history of hypertension and tobacco use is **unable to speak.**
HPI	The patient was well this morning, but during a meeting his speech became slow and then stopped altogether. He was **able to follow instructions** to get up and walk but needed help walking. He was brought to the ER by a colleague. The patient has a history of **hypercholesterolemia.**
PE	VS: normal HR; hypertension (BP 185/95). PE: alert and **able to follow commands** but **unable to repeat commands; nonfluent speech;** able to name two of three objects but unable to name parts of objects; right facial droop; right upper extremity 3/5, and right lower extremity 4/5 on motor exam.
Labs	CBC/Lytes: normal. PT/PTT and glucose normal. ECG: sinus rhythm with LVH.
Imaging	CT-Brain (on admission): no hemorrhage; no mass; no shift. CT-Brain (24 hours later): ischemic **infarct of the left posterior inferior frontal gyrus** (= BROCA'S AREA). US-Carotid: 80% left **ICA stenosis.** Echo: no thrombus.
Pathogenesis	Broca's aphasia is a nonfluent (motor) aphasia characterized by broken speech in which patients are unable to produce spoken language, but **comprehension** of speech **remains intact.** Characteristically, patients are aware of their deficit and are frustrated with their inability to communicate. Hypertension, elevated serum cholesterol, and tobacco use are independent risk factors for the development of ischemic stroke.
Epidemiology	An estimated 500,000 new cases of stroke of all types occur each year; strokes are a common cause of death and disability. Modifiable risk factors include tobacco use, hypertension, diabetes mellitus, and hypercholesterolemia.
Management	**Anti-platelet agent** (e.g, aspirin) for secondary stroke prevention; heparin for DVT prophylaxis. Hold antihypertensive agents for 2–4 weeks, as cerebral hypoperfusion is a risk. Six weeks after stroke, obtain an MR to confirm the extent of ICA stenosis. **Carotid endarterectomy** is indicated if stenosis on symptomatic side is > 70%. Endarterectomy is not indicated until six

weeks after acute stroke.

Complications	Recurrent ischemic infarcts and CAD.
Associated Diseases	◘ **Conduction Aphasia** Disconnection between language centers due to a temporal lobe lesion; presents with fluent, paraphasic speech that is incomprehensible; receptive comprehension intact; CT or MR reveals lesion of temporal lobe; treat with speech therapy.

◘ **Wernicke's Aphasia** A disorder of language comprehension due to a lesion of the posterior superior temporal lobe (= WERNICKE'S AREA); commonly embolic in origin; fluent, paraphasic speech that is empty of meaning (= WORD SALAD); comprehension is impaired; hemiparesis mild or absent; MR or CT may reveal temporal lobe lesion; treat with speech therapy.

ID/CC	A 57-year-old left-handed man complains of acute-onset, **severe headache** and then develops **weakness on the left side of his body** (= HEMIPLEGIA).
HPI	The patient has **hypertension** that has been treated with multiple antihypertensives. Three months ago, he stopped taking all his prescription medications (= NONCOMPLIANT WITH MEDICATIONS). He was asymptomatic until this morning.
PE	VS: **hypertension** (BP 205/110); normal HR. PE: lethargic; responsive to voices but unable to follow commands; positive doll's eyes; left facial droop but able to raise eyebrows (= UPPER MOTOR NEURON LEFT FACIAL PALSY); motor strength 0/5 in left upper and lower extremity; left Babinski's present.
Labs	CBC/Lytes: normal. Glucose normal, PT/PTT and platelets normal. ECG: sinus rhythm with LVH.
Imaging	[A] CT-Head: focal hemorrhage involving the right basal ganglia.
Pathogenesis	The **most common causes** of intracerebral hemorrhage are **hypertension, vascular malformation, tumor,** and **cerebral amyloid angiopathy.** The most common sites of hypertensive hemorrhage are the basal ganglia (putamen and thalamus), cerebellum, and pons.
Epidemiology	Fifteen percent of all strokes are hemorrhagic.
Management	**Intubate** for airway protection; administer **IV beta-blockers to keep systolic BP < 150** (try to reduce blood pressure to the lowest level that can maintain cerebral perfusion). Mechanical hyperventilation and IV mannitol can be used if there is an increase in ICP. These treatments will provide time for surgical intervention to prevent brainstem herniation.
Complications	Complications include **recurrent stroke** and hypertensive encephalopathy. Early mortality rate is higher than observed in infarction. Level of consciousness is a strong prognostic factor. Comatose patients have a mortality rate of approximately 90%.
Associated Diseases	◾ **Thrombotic Stroke** Cerebral infarction caused by local thrombosis secondary to atherosclerosis, vasculitis, hypercoagulable state (e.g., polycythemia, anti-

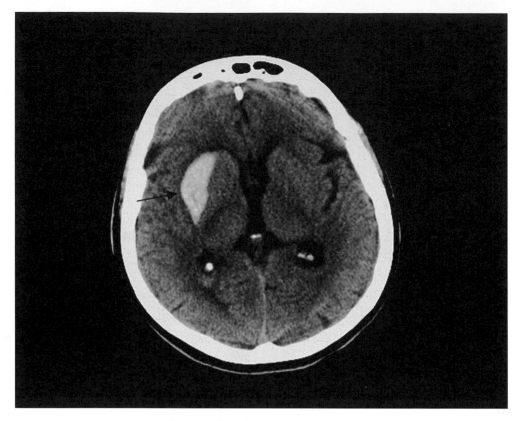

phospholipid syndrome), or cocaine abuse; presents with focal neurologic deficits; head CT or MR demonstrates infarction; treat with tPA if the patient presents within 3 hours of symptom onset and there is no evidence of hemorrhage; heparin is controversial even without evidence of hemorrhage; in the long term, administer aspirin and physical/occupational rehabilitation.

◪ **Lacunar Stroke** Small infarctions most commonly within the basal ganglia, pons, and internal capsule; associated with hypertension and diabetes; presents with contralateral motor or sensory deficit, ataxic hemiparesis, or dysarthria/clumsy hand syndrome; CT shows small, punched-out hypodense lesions; treat by controlling hypertension.

◪ **Pseudobulbar Palsy** A syndrome characterized by bulbar deficits; etiologies include vascular dementia and progressive supranuclear palsy; presents with inappropriate, uncontrollable emotional outbursts (laughing, crying), dysarthria, dysphagia, and hyperactive gag and jaw-jerk reflexes; treat underlying hypertension.

ID/CC	A 74-year-old African-American male with a history of **hypertension** and **non-insulin-dependent diabetes mellitus** (NIDDM) complains of sudden-onset **weakness in his right hand** and **drooling.**
HPI	He was asymptomatic when he went to bed, but when he woke up he noted clumsiness while brushing his teeth. He also noted drooling out of the right side of his mouth.
PE	VS: **hypertension** (BP 175/95). PE: alert and oriented; dysarthria; right facial droop with no forehead weakness (due to UMN right facial nerve palsy); motor strength 4/5 in right arm, 5/5 in right leg, and 5/5 in left arm and leg; reflexes 2+ and symmetric; Babinski's absent; sensory exam normal.
Labs	CBC: normal. Blood glucose elevated; **hypercholesterolemia** (LDL 295 mg/dL). ECG: sinus rhythm with LVH.
Imaging	CT-Brain (on admission): no mass; no shift; no hemorrhage; periventricular white matter disease consistent with small vessel ischemia. CT-Head (24 hours after admission): lacunar ischemic infarct in the posterior limb of the left internal capsule (due to involvement of thalamoperforate arteries). [A] CT-Head: another case showing bilateral lacunar infarcts. US-Carotid: no significant stenosis. Echo: no thrombus; LVH.
Pathogenesis	Lacunar infarcts are caused by occlusion of penetrating branches of the circle of Willis, MCA, or vertebral and basilar arteries due to thrombosis or lipohyalinotic thickening of these branches.
Epidemiology	Lacunar strokes account for approximately 20% of all strokes.
Management	**Anti-platelet agents** (e.g., aspirin, ticlopidine) reduce stroke risk by 25%; begin after the initial head CT has ruled out cerebral hemorrhage. **Heparin** is given for DVT prophylaxis and **lipid-lowering drugs** are given to reduce the risk of further strokes. Physical and occupational therapy are often useful in achieving maximal function.
Complications	Lacunar stroke patients have a 15% chance of recurrence

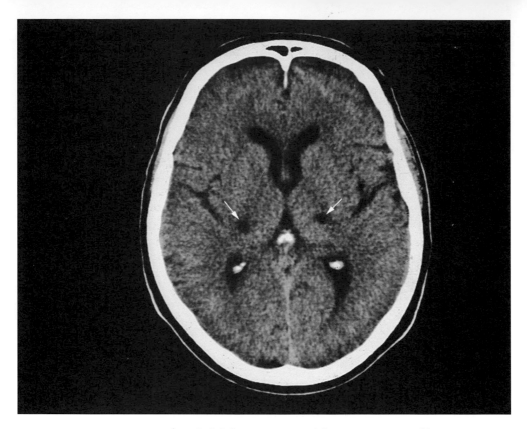

after initial recovery with an 8% mortality rate.

Associated Diseases

☐ **Thrombotic Stroke** Cerebral infarction caused by local thrombosis secondary to atherosclerosis, vasculitis, hypercoagulable state (e.g., polycythemia, anti-phospholipid syndrome), or cocaine abuse; presents with focal neurologic deficits; head CT or MR demonstrates infarction; treat with tPA if the patient presents within three hours of symptom onset and there is no evidence of hemorrhage; heparin is controversial even without evidence of hemorrhage; in the longer term, administer aspirin and physical/occupational rehabilitation.

ID/CC	A 91-year-old right-handed woman is found on the floor **unable to speak or move the right side of her body.**
HPI	The patient lives alone and was last seen two days ago. The woman was grunting and not moving her right side.
PE	VS: **hypotension** (BP 80/50); **irregularly irregular pulse** (due to atrial fibrillation; average HR 110). PE: alert; unable to speak spontaneously or to repeat or follow commands; motor strength 0/5 in right arm and leg with Babinski's present; reflexes 2+ and symmetric; no cranial nerve palsies.
Labs	CBC normal. Elevated BUN (55 mg/dL); normal creatinine (1.1 mg/dL) (prerenal azotemia due to dehydration or low cardiac output). Lytes: normal. ECG: **atrial fibrillation** with fast ventricular rate.
Imaging	**[A]** CT-Head: hypodensity (1) involving the entire left MCA distribution (classic sign of completed ischemic infarct). Echo: no thrombus; dilated left atrium; LV ejection fraction of 55%.
Pathogenesis	Left MCA occlusion causes **contralateral hemiplegia, hemisensory loss,** and **loss of right visual field** (= HOMONYMOUS HEMIANOPSIA). The inability to speak, repeat, and understand language (= GLOBAL APHASIA) results when the dominant hemisphere is involved, including Broca's area, Wernicke's area, and the arcuate fasciculus.
Epidemiology	The annual risk of stroke with atrial fibrillation is 5%.
Management	Prevent recurrent strokes in those with atrial fibrillation by placing on **long-term anticoagulation with warfarin.** For maximal recovery after this event, physical, occupational, and speech therapy are necessary.
Complications	The most common complications are pneumonia and UTI due to Foley catheterization. Other complications include hemorrhagic transformation of the ischemic infarct and recurrent infarcts. Left MCA infarction also causes aphasia, alexia, agraphia, acalculia, and right/left confusion in addition to right-sided hemiplegia. **FIRST AID 2** p. 234
Associated Diseases	N/A

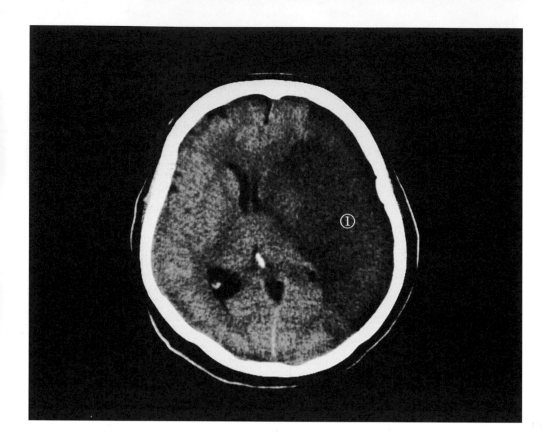

ID/CC	A 55-year-old right-handed female with **chronic hypertension** presents with **acute-onset left-sided weakness** and **altered sensorium.**
HPI	The patient is being treated for hypertension. This morning, her husband found her on the floor next to the bed unable to move her left arm and leg. She could speak but was "acting funny."
PE	VS: **hypertension** (BP 180/100). PE: alert with fluent speech; answers questions appropriately but is **unable to draw a clock or copy a five-sided figure correctly; eyes deviated to right; 0/5 strength in left arm and leg** and 5/5 strength in right arm and leg; DTRs 2+ in right arm and leg and 3+ in left arm and leg; increased tone in left arm and leg, normal in right arm and leg; Babinski's present on left; no carotid or subclavian bruit; no cardiac murmurs.
Labs	CBC/Lytes: normal. PT/PTT and glucose normal. Lytes: normal. VDRL negative; antiphospholipid antibodies negative; elevated cholesterol and triglycerides.
Imaging	CT-Head (within 24 hours): no mass, hemorrhage, or midline shift. **[A]** CT-Head (after 48 hours): right MCA infarct with extensive hypodensity (1). **[B]** MR-Brain: another patient with a smaller T2-hyperintense right MCA infarct.
Pathogenesis	Hypertension is an independent risk factor for the development of ischemic stroke. Right MCA occlusion causes **contralateral hemiplegia, hemisensory loss,** and **loss of left visual field** (= HOMONYMOUS HEMIANOPIA) with **deviation of the eyes to the side of the lesion.** There is also global aphasia if the dominant hemisphere is affected.
Epidemiology	There are 500,000 new strokes each year in the U.S. Strokes are a common cause of disability. Modifiable risk factors include **tobacco use, hypertension, diabetes mellitus,** and **hypercholesterolemia.**
Management	**Anti-platelet agents** reduce stroke risk by 25%; begin them after the initial head CT has ruled out cerebral hemorrhage. **Lipid-lowering drugs** also reduce the risk of recurrent stroke.

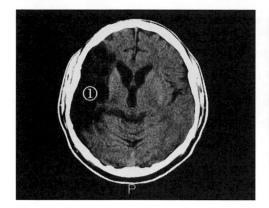 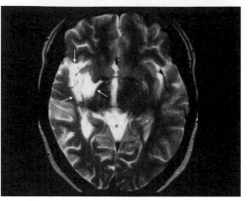

Complications   Complications include recurrent stroke, MI, DVT, UTI, and aspiration pneumonia. Loss of consciousness renders a poorer prognosis.

Associated Diseases   N/A

ID/CC	A 42-year-old **woman** presents with **left facial droop** and **left hemiparesis** following a seizure.
HPI	According to a witness, she complained of the acute onset of a severe, **"worst-ever" headache** followed by nausea and vomiting. Shortly thereafter she had a seizure and was then lethargic.
PE	VS: tachycardia (HR 112); slight fever (37.8 C). PE: moaning, irritable, and confused; **decerebrate posturing;** depressed level of consciousness; **nuchal rigidity; Kernig's and Brudzinski's signs positive; left facial droop; left hemiplegia; left hyperreflexia;** funduscopy reveals **papilledema.**
Labs	CBC: normal. Lytes: hyponatremia (due to SIADH). PT/PTT normal (rules out SAH due to blood dyscrasias). ECG: inverted T waves (= ROLLER COASTER T WAVES). LP: not done, since CT provides clear evidence of SAH.
Imaging	**[A]** CT-Head: hyperdensity (1) in the right MCA region representing hemorrhage from a ruptured aneurysm, with bilateral hyperdensities in sulci consistent with SAH. **[B]** CT-Head: another SAH with the circle of Willis outlined by hyperdense subarachnoid blood.
Pathogenesis	The most common cause of spontaneous SAH is **ruptured berry aneurysm.** Aneurysms (which can be seen in **[C]** an angiogram) develop because of a congenital weakness at **points of bifurcation in the circle of Willis.**
Epidemiology	Shows slight female predominance.
Management	Seizure prophylaxis with phenytoin and the calcium channel blocker **nimodipine** to prevent vasospasm. Obtain a cerebral angiogram of all four vessels as soon as possible. **Surgery** should be performed within 48 hours to ensure maximal recovery. Patients with serious neurologic deficits do not benefit from early surgery. Aneurysms > 7 mm require prophylactic surgery. Hydrocephalus requires ventriculostomy or ventriculoperitoneal shunting.
Complications	**Vasospasm** (most common cause of death) leads to

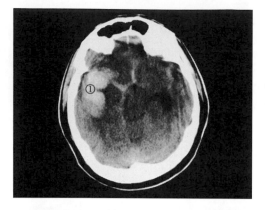
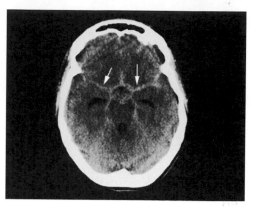
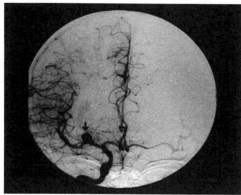

infarction of surrounding tissue; blood in the subarachnoid space or cerebral cortex acts as a **seizure** focus. Other complications include cranial nerve palsies (most commonly CN III), **hydrocephalus,** high-protein pulmonary edema, rebleed, and severe hyponatremia due to SIADH. **FIRST AID 2** p. 225

Associated Diseases

◻ **AV Malformation** Congenital vascular malformations, more common in men; CNS AVMs present with headache and seizures; contrast CT, angiography, and MR reveal AVM; treat with coiling, surgical excision or embolization; complications include rupture causing intracerebral or subarachnoid bleed.

◻ **Epidural Hematoma** Collection of blood between the dura mater and skull due to rupture of the middle meningeal artery; presents with headache, confusion with lucid intervals, weakness, blurry vision, and projectile vomiting; CT shows a convex, lens-shaped, hyperdense extra-axial fluid collection; treat with emergent surgical evacuation.

21.

CVA – SUBARACHNOID HEMORRHAGE

ID/CC	A 62-year-old right-handed female with a history of **paroxysmal atrial tachycardia** is brought to the hospital after "not making sense" at work.
HPI	The patient was at a meeting when she suddenly began **speaking "gibberish."** She was **unable to follow instructions** to get up. However, once her colleague helped her up, she was able to walk to the car without assistance.
PE	VS: **hypertension** (BP 160/100); **pulse irregularly irregular.** PE: alert and in no acute distress with clear but unintelligible speech (= FLUENT APHASIA); **unable to repeat phrases** or follow commands; **paraphasic errors** (e.g., "shoon" instead of "spoon") and **neologisms** (nonexistent words, e.g., "bork"); cranial nerves intact; motor strength 5/5 and DTRs 2+ throughout; Babinski's absent.
Labs	CBC: normal. ECG: atrial fibrillation with controlled ventricular rate. Lytes: normal. PT/PTT and glucose normal.
Imaging	CT-Head (on admission): no mass; no hemorrhage; no infarct. CT-Head (24 hours after admission): ischemic infarct in the left superior temporal gyrus. US-Carotid: no hemodynamically significant stenosis. Echo: dilated left atrium; no thrombus.
Pathogenesis	Wernicke's aphasia is typically due to a **cardioembolic event.** Typically, patients are unaware that their speech is incomprehensible.
Epidemiology	The annual risk of stroke with atrial fibrillation is 5%.
Management	The patient with atrial fibrillation should be placed on **lifelong anticoagulation** with **warfarin** as well as **antiplatelet** agents to reduce the risk of stroke recurrence. Speech therapy is useful.
Complications	Recurrent stroke and MI.
Associated Diseases	◼ **Broca's Aphasia** A disorder of language production caused by a lesion of the dominant inferior frontal gyrus (= BROCA'S AREA); presents with nonfluent, labored, dysarthric speech, intact comprehension, associated hemiparesis, and apraxia of oral muscles; treat with speech therapy.

◻ **Conduction Aphasia** Disconnection between language centers due to a temporal lobe lesion; presents with fluent, paraphasic speech that is incomprehensible; receptive comprehension intact; CT or MR reveals lesion of temporal lobe; treat with speech therapy.

ID/CC	An **82-year-old** woman with dementia who resides at a nursing home presents with a change in mental status.
HPI	The patient was in her usual state of health at dinner the previous night. In the morning, she was unable to get out of bed and was unable to speak.
PE	VS: no fever; **hypertension** (BP 160/95). PE: alert but unable to follow simple commands; unable to state her name (= APHASIA); right facial droop noted; motor strength 5/5 throughout; reflexes 2+ and symmetric; Babinski's absent.
Labs	CBC/Lytes: normal. PT/PTT, glucose, BUN, and creatinine normal.
Imaging	**[A]** CT-Head: cortical hemorrhage in the left frontal lobe (1).
Pathogenesis	Cerebral amyloid angiopathy (CAA) is characterized by **deposition of amyloid in small and medium-sized arteries in the cortex.** It may result in one or multiple simultaneous intracerebral, subarachnoid, or lobar hemorrhages. Clinical dementia is seen in 10%–30% of patients with CAA. Pathologically, 50% present with neuritic plaques. The characteristic lesion is **Congo-red-positive, apple-green, birefringent** amyloid in the media and adventitia of arteries.
Epidemiology	**Incidence increases with age;** seen in 60% of autopsies in those > 90 years old.
Management	IV **beta-blockers** to keep systolic BP < 150.
Complications	Recurrent stroke.
Associated Diseases	N/A

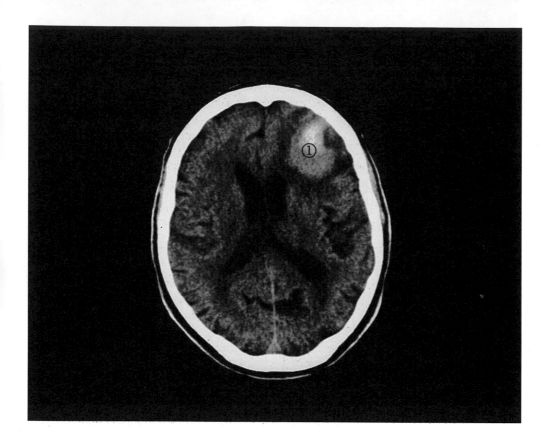

CVA DUE TO AMYLOID ANGIOPATHY

ID/CC	A **76-year-old** female is brought in because she **has not been able to concentrate or think clearly** while playing cards; she has also had **trouble recalling recent events** in her life for approximately one month.
HPI	Her daughter states that for the past six months she has observed changes in her mother's behavior, including **bizarre acts** and an **inability to recall recent events** (often the first symptom).
PE	VS: normal. PE: in no acute distress; awake, alert, and oriented to time, space, and person; speech normal, but at times content and form are not appropriate; impaired immediate and recent memory; pupils equal, round, and reactive to light and accommodation; extraocular muscles intact; no abnormal movements; no focal neurologic defects.
Labs	CBC/Lytes/LFTs: normal. Glucose and TFTs normal. UA: normal.
Imaging	**[A]** CT-Head: cerebral atrophy with ventricular dilatation.
Pathogenesis	A degenerative neurologic disease of unknown etiology, it is associated with cholinergic deficiency and is characterized by the development of dementia. **Abnormal neuronal membrane metabolism of phospholipids** has been implicated as a pathogenic mechanism, as has aluminum toxicity. **Neurofibrillary tangles, amyloid-containing neuritic plaques, diffuse cortical atrophy,** and **ventricular dilatation** are the characteristic pathologic findings.
Epidemiology	Alzheimer's disease is the most common cause of dementia; **70% of all cases of senile dementia** are caused by Alzheimer's and 20% by multi-infarct dementia. The incidence of Alzheimer's increases with advancing age. Most patients with Down's syndrome develop Alzheimer's by age 40.
Management	Treatment is largely **supportive.** Discontinue drugs that exacerbate disorientation and confusion (sedatives, anxiolytics); treat concomitant disorders (infections, endocrine problems). The cholinesterase inhibitor tacrine may be tried (side effect is liver toxicity) but is most useful in mild to moderate cases. Donepezil

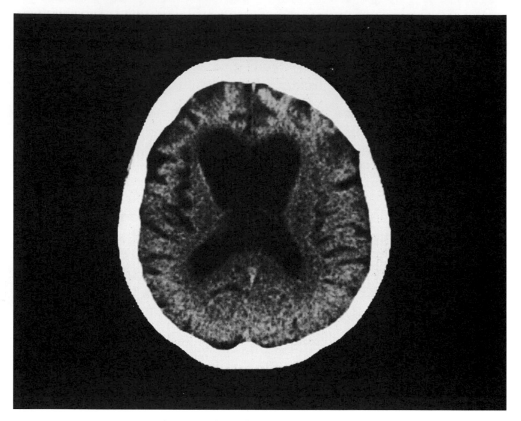

(Aricept) is also potentially useful.

Complications Disability, disorientation, social withdrawal, confusion, pneumonia, and suicide.

Associated Diseases ◘ **Multi-infarct Dementia** The second most common cause of dementia (after Alzheimer's disease); associated with hypertension; presents with stepwise progression of dementia; patients may have pathologic emotionality (= PSEUDOBULBAR EFFECT); CT/MR may show multiple subcortical infarcts; treat by controlling hypertension and cholesterol to reduce the risk of further infarctions.

◘ **Normal Pressure Communicating Hydrocephalus** Idiopathic or secondary to compromised CSF absorption (meningitis, SAH); presents with dementia, gait ataxia, and incontinence; CT/MR show enlarged lateral ventricles; treat with lumbar-peritoneal shunt.

◘ **Down's Syndrome** The most common chromosomal disorder; due to trisomy 21; higher incidence in advancing maternal age; older patients with Down's syndrome are predisposed to Alzheimer's dementia;

presents as developmentally retarded neonate with classic Down's facies (epicanthal folds, low-set ears, macroglossia), hypotonia, and simian crease; karyotype reveals trisomy 21; prenatal diagnosis is possible by chromosomal analysis of chorionic villous biopsy or amniocentesis and decreased levels of maternal serum alpha-fetoprotein levels; treatment consists of social service support; common complications include leukemia and heart disease.

ID/CC   An **81-year-old** right-handed **male** with a history of insulin-dependent diabetes mellitus (IDDM) and **hypertension** presents with gradually progressing confusion over the past several years.

HPI   He has had two strokes with residual left hemiparesis; he was brought to the hospital by his wife due to **increasing confusion** and **angry outbursts.** He has forgotten important appointments, repeatedly **asks the same questions,** and **forgets names** (all due to memory impairment). He has also become irritable, easily frustrated, and suspicious and demanding of his wife (all due to behavioral impairment). For the past two years he has not driven a car because he becomes confused at intersections. He has recently been **getting lost** when he takes walks (due to visual and spatial disorientation).

PE   VS: **hypertension** (BP 150/90). PE: pleasant and alert; **oriented to person only;** speech fluent; **cannot recall current President or recent news events,** and **cannot perform mathematical calculations** (serial sevens, simple addition and subtraction); mild left facial droop; 4/5 strength in left upper and lower extremities with mild increase in tone; 5/5 strength in right upper and lower extremities; DTRs 3+ in left upper and lower extremities and 2+ in right upper and lower extremities; **positive snout and palmar-mental reflexes** (= PRIMITIVE REFLEXES); **Babinski's present bilaterally** (sign of global hemispheric dysfunction); withdraws to pain in all four extremities; finger-to-nose intact bilaterally.

Labs   CBC: normal. Serum VDRL, TFTs, B_{12}, and folate levels normal. EEG: moderate to marked generalized slowing; no epileptiform activity.

Imaging   CT-Head: diffuse **periventricular hypodensity;** small old ischemic infarcts; no hemorrhage; no mass.

Pathogenesis   An accumulation of defects from **multiple, bilateral cerebral infarcts.** Patients with previous cerebral insults will have reduced cerebral reserve and are more vulnerable to confusion from minor insults. Dementia can be classified as cortical or subcortical. **Cortical** causes include primary degenerative dementias like Alzheimer's, Pick's disease, Creutzfeldt–Jacob disease, multi-infarct dementia, and dementias due to other causes such as normal pressure hydrocephalus, mass lesions, drugs, and HIV. **Subcortical** dementias include Parkinson's and Huntington's dementia.

Epidemiology Causes 15%–30% of all dementias; typically occurs in **patients > 50 years** with a **history of generalized atherosclerotic disease. Men** are affected more often than women.

Management Aggressive **control of hypertension** to prevent further decline. Medium-potency **neuroleptics** such as thioridazine may be administered for control of aggressive behavior.

Complications Urinary incontinence, seizure disorder (infarcted regions can serve as a seizure focus), and dysphagia resulting in aspiration pneumonia.

Associated Diseases ◘ **Alzheimer's Disease** A slowly progressive, degenerative brain disease; the most common cause of dementia; presents with insidious global cognitive decline; pathologic findings include beta-amyloid plaques and neurofibrillary tangles; treat with social services to aid the family in the patient's care; tacrine may slow decline in cognition.

◘ **Delirium** An acute fluctuating confusional state with global attention impairment secondary to systemic problems (e.g., drugs, sepsis, metabolic imbalances); presents with waxing and waning levels of consciousness, perceptual disturbances, and delusions; treat the underlying cause; can administer haloperidol or benzodiazepines for sedation.

◘ **Pseudodementia** A cognitive dysfunction resulting from depression; reversible and common; screen for depression; treat with SSRIs.

ID/CC	A 33-year-old woman who **recently had a URI** now complains of **loss of strength in her lower legs** and difficulty walking.
HPI	Over the past four weeks, she has noted **symmetric weakness** starting in her lower limbs and progressing to her hips and upper limbs (= ASCENDING PARALYSIS). Over the past week she has experienced occasional urinary incontinence, lightheadedness on rising quickly, and shortness of breath.
PE	VS: no fever; **orthostatic hypotension; tachycardia** (due to autonomic dysfunction). PE: mental status normal; marked symmetric **loss of motor strength** with **flaccidity** most notable in **proximal lower limbs; absent patellar and Achilles reflexes bilaterally;** mild facial weakness.
Labs	LP: **elevated protein in CSF; normal cellularity** (= CYTOALBUMINIC DISSOCIATION). Serum B_{12} normal; FTA negative; glucose normal. Lytes: normal. EMG: markedly slowed motor and sensory conduction. Nerve conduction studies reveal evidence of **demyelination** with **slowing of conduction velocity** and multifocal conduction blocks.
Imaging	CT/MR-Brain: No intracranial lesions or hemorrhage.
Pathogenesis	An acute demyelinating polyradiculoneuropathy that is believed to be an **autoimmune-mediated reaction** to certain infectious agents. The most common pathogens are thought to be *Campylobacter jejuni,* viral hepatitis, and EBV. Guillain–Barré syndrome can also occur following influenza vaccinations.
Epidemiology	There is a bimodal age distribution, with most cases occurring in early adulthood or between 45 and 64 years. There is no known HLA association.
Management	**Plasmapheresis** is the treatment of choice. Patients with hemodynamic instability and children may be given **IV immunoglobulin.** Hospitalization for potential respiratory failure (and subsequent mechanical ventilation).
Complications	Can lead to **respiratory insufficiency** that may require ventilatory support. Recovery is complete in approximately 50%; 40% have mild disability, and 10%

GUILLAIN–BARRÉ SYNDROME

have severe permanent disability. Mortality arises from cardiac arrhythmias or superimposed viral or bacterial pneumonia.

<table>
<tr><td>Associated Diseases</td><td>

■ **Botulism** Flaccid paralysis due to botulinum toxin; inhibits the release of acetylcholine at the neuromuscular junction; seen in adults after the ingestion of toxin in home-canned goods; seen in infants after the ingestion of spores in contaminated honey; presents with double vision, weakness, cranial nerve palsies, and progressive respiratory failure; toxin is detected in serum; treat with antitoxin; intubate to support ventilation.

■ **Myasthenia Gravis** A neuromuscular disease caused by autoantibodies against acetylcholine receptors, associated with thymomas; presents with fatigue and muscle weakness made worse by exercise; improves with rest; ocular symptoms such as diplopia are especially prominent; administration of acetylcholinesterase inhibitors temporarily ameliorates symptoms; treat with pyridostigmine; thymectomy improves symptoms in 50% of patients.
</td></tr>
</table>

GUILLAIN–BARRÉ SYNDROME

ID/CC	A 52-year-old male presents with **left eyelid droop** (= PTOSIS) and **lack of perspiration** on the left side (= ANHIDROSIS) following a motor vehicle accident.
HPI	The patient has no significant medical history. He was "rear-ended" at a traffic light.
PE	VS: normal. PE: **left pupil constricted** (= MIOSIS); left eyelid drooping; perspiration palpable on right side of forehead but not on left.
Labs	CBC: normal. PT/PTT normal.
Imaging	US-Carotid: occlusion of the left internal carotid artery consistent with carotid dissection.
Pathogenesis	The course of the **sympathetic tract** can be disrupted at a number of sites, causing Horner's syndrome. The syndrome may be caused by any lesion that disrupts the sympathetic fibers in the carotid plexus, cervical sympathetic chain, upper thoracic cord (e.g., superior sulcus or Pancoast's lung tumors), or brainstem (Wallenberg's syndrome).
Epidemiology	The syndrome is relatively rare.
Management	Manage these patients in the **ICU.** When the cause of Horner's is carotid dissection, IV **heparin** and 3–6 months of **warfarin** is the accepted treatment. Prevention of unequal pupils is impossible.
Complications	N/A
Associated Diseases	◘ **Pseudobulbar Palsy** A syndrome characterized by bulbar deficits; etiologies include vascular dementia and progressive supranuclear palsy; presents with inappropriate, uncontrollable emotional outbursts (laughing, crying), dysarthria, dysphagia, and hyperactive gag and jaw-jerk reflexes; treat underlying hypertension to prevent new infarcts. ◘ **Bell's Palsy** The most common form of facial paralysis; idiopathic; rapid onset of usually unilateral facial weakness; treat with eye protection; a short corticosteroid course may speed recovery.

ID/CC	A **35-year-old** male presents with **episodes** of **nausea** and **dizziness** of one month's duration.
HPI	At first the patient had episodes of nausea and a sensation that the "room was spinning" (= VERTIGO); these episodes lasted 3–5 minutes. Over the past week, however, the symptoms have persisted for 1–2 hours. A severe episode two days ago resulted in emesis and "buzzing" in the left ear (= TINNITUS).
PE	VS: normal. PE: mild sensorineural hearing loss in left ear; **Bárány maneuver** fails to reproduce sensation of vertigo; remainder of neurologic exam normal.
Labs	CBC: normal. Serum VDRL negative.
Imaging	MR-Brain: unremarkable.
Pathogenesis	The condition is caused by an **increase in volume of the endolymphatic system** (= ENDOLYMPHATIC HYDROPS), resulting in distention. The primary lesion is thought to be in the endolymphatic sac, which is responsible for endolymph filtration and excretion. Two known causes are syphilis and head trauma.
Epidemiology	Typical onset is in middle age.
Management	Treat acute attacks with **bed rest; meclizine** or **dimenhydrinate** are used for symptomatic relief of vertigo. Chronic treatment involves institution of a **low-sodium diet** and **diuretics.** To treat intractable disease, a **surgical shunt** should be placed (relieves vertigo in 70% but causes hearing loss in 50% of cases).
Complications	**Remissions and relapses** may occur throughout life; gradual **hearing loss** due to multiple attacks is possible.
Associated Diseases	◘ **Acute Labyrinthitis** May result from viral or bacterial infections; typically self-limiting; presents with abrupt onset of severe continuous vertigo, tinnitus, and hearing loss; treat with bed rest, vestibular suppressants, and avoidance of rapid head movements.
	◘ **Acoustic Neuroma** A vestibular nerve schwannoma (if bilateral, suspect neurofibromatosis type 2); presents with features of cerebellopontine angle compression and vestibulo-auditory impairment (tinnitus, vertigo, and hearing loss); CT/MR show an enhancing

cerebellopontine angle mass with an enlarged internal acoustic meatus; radiation therapy or surgical resection is curative.

◘ **Benign Positional Vertigo** A common form of vertigo resulting from a dislodged fragment of otolith in the semicircular canals; presents with transient episodic vertigo associated with changes in position; treat with repositioning exercises.

ID/CC	A **30-year-old woman** complains of gradual diminution of vision in the right eye.
HPI	She has had several **prior neurologic symptoms,** including an episode of loss of sensation and tingling in her left leg one year ago that lasted 2–3 days; she did not seek medical attention at that time. She has noted a gradual decrease of vision in her right eye over the last week with discomfort on moving the right eye.
PE	VS: normal. PE: nystagmus; unable to adduct eyes on lateral gaze (internuclear ophthalmoplegia); swollen right optic nerve (due to optic neuritis) with blurred margins; visual acuity 20/400 in right eye and 20/20 in left eye; DTRs asymmetrically hyperactive; sensory and cerebellar exam intact.
Labs	LP: CSF shows **lymphocytic pleocytosis, oligoclonal bands** (most specific lab abnormality), elevated myelin basic protein, and negative Lyme titer. Impaired visual, auditory, and somatosensory evoked responses.
Imaging	**[A]** MR-Brain: **multiple periventricular white matter lesions** on T2-weighted image. **[B]** MR-Spine: large hyperintense plaque of demyelination at C5 level.
Pathogenesis	Probably an autoimmune process triggered by a virus (via molecular mimicry) occurring in a genetically susceptible person. The specific pathology is **demyelination** with axonal sparing. Any area of the CNS may be involved, but lesions commonly occur in the **lateral ventricular margins** of the **fourth ventricle.**
Epidemiology	Mean age of onset is 32 years with a female to male ratio of 3 to 2; 25% have a **family history.** Frequency rate **declines with increasing proximity to the equator.**
Management	Seventy percent of cases remit spontaneously. **Beta-interferon** may be given to prevent recurrences in patients with relapsing MS. Corticosteroids are used for the treatment of acute relapses. Anticholinergics are given for urinary frequency and urgency; baclofen is useful in treating spasticity. Nocturnal spasms can be relieved by diazepam, and diffuse dysesthetic pain responds to carbamazepine or gabapentin.
Complications	As the disease progresses there is increased motor tone

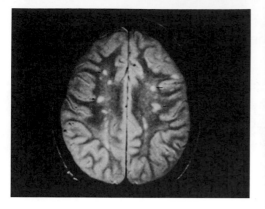

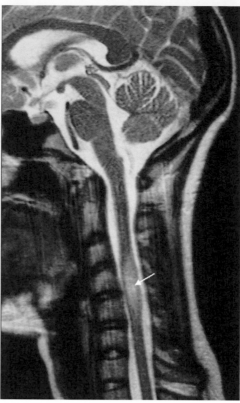

and spasticity, bladder dysfunction, and fatigue.

Associated Diseases   N/A

ID/CC	A **40-year-old woman** complains of **occasional double vision** and "**droopy**" **eyelids**.
HPI	For the past three months, she has noted intermittent diplopia that arises when she is watching television. Her husband adds that her **eyelids become droopy at night but are normal in the morning.**
PE	VS: normal. PE: **bilateral ptosis** that **worsens with repeated blinking;** extraocular muscles intact with diplopia on extremes of lateral gaze; motor strength 5/5 bilaterally on initial and 4/5 on prolonged testing; DTRs normal; sensory exam normal.
Labs	**Elevated acetylcholine receptor antibody** titer. EMG: decrease in muscle action potential with repeated firing. **Tensilon** test (IV injection of acetylcholinesterase inhibitor) leads to resolution of ptosis and diplopia on lateral gaze.
Imaging	**[A]** CT-Chest: lobular **thymic mass** in the anterior mediastinum.
Pathogenesis	An **autoimmune process.** Antibodies are produced to the acetylcholine receptor, resulting in the destruction of receptors and disruption of the neuromuscular junction. Can be distinguished clinically from Eaton–Lambert syndrome by **worsening rather than improving symptoms with repetitive motion.**
Epidemiology	Myasthenia gravis has a prevalence of approximately 1 in 7,000 with a peak incidence in younger women and older men.
Management	**Pyridostigmine,** a cholinesterase inhibitor, is used for symptomatic relief of weakness. Long-term **immunosuppression** with corticosteroids and azathioprine. Treat acute exacerbations with **plasmapheresis** and IV **immunoglobulin. Thymectomy** may help up to 85% of patients.
Complications	**Myasthenic crisis** is typically an acute exacerbation involving respiratory muscles that may require mechanical ventilation; it is often secondary to underlying infection.
Associated Diseases	◻ **Botulism** Flaccid paralysis due to botulinum toxin; inhibits the release of acetylcholine at the neuromuscular

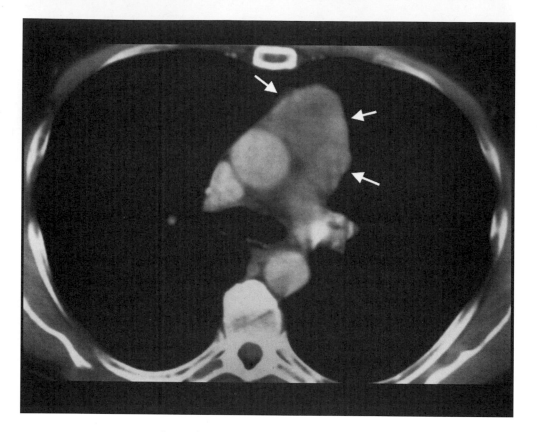

junction; seen in adults after the ingestion of toxin in home-canned goods; seen in infants after the ingestion of spores in contaminated honey; presents with double vision, weakness, cranial nerve palsies, and progressive respiratory failure; toxin is detected in serum; treat with antitoxin; intubate to support ventilation.

■ **Eaton–Lambert Syndrome** A paraneoplastic myasthenia-like syndrome due to antibodies directed at presynaptic calcium ion channels at the neuromuscular junction; presents with weakness (usually proximal) and autonomic dysfunction; EMG shows diagnostic increase in action potential with repetitive stimulation; treat with corticosteroids or plasmapheresis; treat underlying carcinoma.

ID/CC	A 34-year-old male presents with **clumsiness of the hands** and multiple "falls."
HPI	The patient is an only child whose **mother died from a "heart attack"** at the age of 40. He has had increasing difficulty using tools, buttoning shirts, and tying his shoes. He has also begun to trip on the rugs at home. He has **difficulty releasing his grip** when shaking hands.
PE	VS: normal. PE: marked male-pattern **baldness; bilateral ptosis** with hollowing of masseter and temples (= HATCHET FACE) and **bilateral facial weakness** (= FISH MOUTH); percussion of thenar eminence produces abduction of thumb and firm contraction of thenar eminence (= MYOTONIA); bilateral foot drop; weakness and difficulty relaxing distal muscles; sensory exam normal; DTRs reduced.
Labs	CBC: normal. Mildly elevated CK; **DNA analysis** reveals 100 copies of a **trinucleotide repeat in the myotonin gene.** EMG: **myotonic discharges.** Muscle biopsy reveals increased number of central nuclei, prominent ring fibers, and areas of disorganized sarcoplasm devoid of normal striations. ECG: **first-degree heart block.**
Imaging	N/A
Pathogenesis	Myotonic dystrophy is inherited as an **autosomal-dominant** disorder. The defect consists of greater than 30 copies of a trinucleotide repeat in the myotonin gene; the function of the myotonin protein is, however, unknown. **Anticipation,** the phenomenon in which successive generations experience more severe disease, is due to expansion in the number of trinucleotide repeats from one generation to the next.
Epidemiology	Incidence is 13.5 in 100,000 live births. The most common muscular dystrophy seen among adults.
Management	Administer **phenytoin** or quinine to relieve myotonia. Use orthotic devices to alleviate foot drop. **Cardiac evaluation** should be performed owing to the high incidence of arrhythmias.
Complications	**Sudden death** due to cardiac conduction defects; cataracts; and testicular atrophy.

....

31.   **MYOTONIC DYSTROPHY**

Associated Diseases

■ **Duchenne's Muscular Dystrophy** An X-linked recessive mutation in the dystrophin gene; onset is by 2–6 years; the most common and lethal muscular dystrophy; presents with clumsiness, waddling gait, pushing off the ground with the hands in order to stand (= GOWERS' MANEUVER), and pseudohypertrophy of calf muscles; CK elevated; replacement of muscle with fibrofatty tissue on biopsy; immunostain for dystrophin expression is diagnostic; there is no effective treatment; death is inevitable by the 20s or 30s (secondary to respiratory failure).

31. MYOTONIC DYSTROPHY

ID/CC	A 72-year-old male presents with **memory loss, gait difficulty,** and **urinary incontinence.**
HPI	He was brought to the physician's office by his wife, who states that over the past year he has become increasingly forgetful. She adds that he has also wet his pants and their bed on several occasions (= URINARY INCONTINENCE). For the past six months, the patient has fallen on numerous occasions and has had difficulty walking in his own home. He has a history of hypertension.
PE	VS: normal. PE: no speech defects; impaired short-term memory; unable to demonstrate how to comb his hair (impaired apraxia); motor strength 5/5 bilaterally throughout; DTRs 2+; gait characterized by short steps; patient can walk only 10 feet before having to sit down.
Labs	Serum B_{12}, folate, and TSH normal; VDRL negative. LP: **opening pressure of 120 mm H_2O;** slightly elevated glucose and protein; no nucleated cells. After 40 mL of CSF was removed, gait improved.
Imaging	[A] CT-Head: **enlarged lateral ventricles** with comparatively normal sulci; periventricular white matter disease consistent with small vessel ischemia; no mass, hemorrhage, or midline shift.
Pathogenesis	The etiology is not known; it is likely due to decreased absorption of CSF across the arachnoid villi.
Epidemiology	N/A
Management	**Large-volume LP** often results in improvement. Approximately one-third of patients improve following placement of a **ventricular shunt.**
Complications	N/A
Associated Diseases	◻ **Alzheimer's Disease** A slowly progressive, degenerative brain disease; the most common cause of dementia; presents with insidious global cognitive decline; pathologic findings include beta-amyloid plaques and neurofibrillary tangles; treat with social services to aid the family in the patient's care; tacrine may slow decline in cognition.

....

32.   **NORMAL PRESSURE HYDROCEPHALUS**

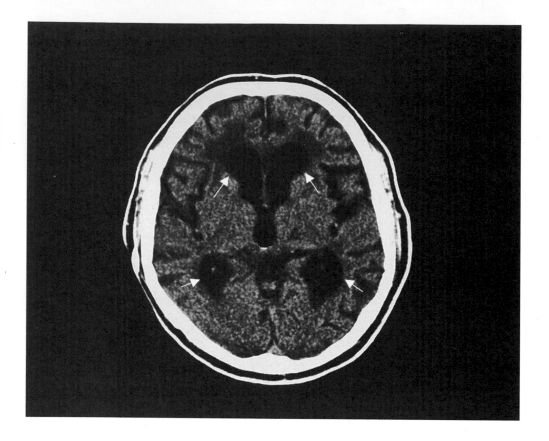

◘ **Multi-infarct Dementia** The second most common cause of dementia (after Alzheimer's disease); associated with hypertension; presents with stepwise progression of dementia; patients may have pathologic emotionality (= PSEUDOBULBAR EFFECT); CT/MR may show multiple subcortical infarcts; treat by controlling hypertension and cholesterol to reduce the risk of further infarctions.

◘ **Parkinson's Disease** Idiopathic destruction of dopaminergic neurons in the substantia nigra; presents with resting tremor ("pill rolling"), flat affect, cogwheel rigidity, akinesis, and postural instability; treat with dopaminergic agonists (levodopa, bromocriptine), MAO-B inhibitors (selegiline), cholinergic antagonists, and amantadine.

NORMAL PRESSURE HYDROCEPHALUS

ID/CC	A **65-year-old** male complains of the development of a **hand tremor** coupled with **generalized muscle rigidity.**
HPI	His wife has noted generalized slowing of movement (= BRADYKINESIA) and **lack of facial expression** (= MASKLIKE FACIES) together with drooling. He has also noticed that his handwriting has been getting smaller (= MICROGRAPHIA). The involuntary tremor decreases during voluntary motion.
PE	VS: normal. PE: severe seborrhea of scalp; sustained blinking follows tapping on nasal bridge (= MYERSON'S SIGN); **postural instability; gait short- and slow-stepped** at first, followed by quick forward steps to prevent fall (= FESTINANT GAIT) with no arm swing; intermittent muscle spasms with passive movement of joints (= COGWHEEL RIGIDITY); DTRs normal; flexor plantar responses.
Labs	ESR normal. Lytes/LFTs: normal. TSH normal.
Imaging	CXR/KUB: within normal limits.
Pathogenesis	Characterized by **loss of dopaminergic neurons in the basal ganglia ([A]** substantia nigra, showing normal population of large pigmented cells; **[B]** severe depletion of pigmented cells), specifically the substantia nigra, which shows loss of pigmentation on postmortem analysis. It is usually idiopathic but may also occur after influenza infections, following carbon monoxide or manganese poisoning, after exposure to the drug **MPTP** (an impurity found in poorly synthesized heroin), with antipsychotic drugs, with basal ganglia tumors, following trauma, and after episodes of encephalitis (= POSTENCEPHALITIC PARKINSONISM).
Epidemiology	A common disorder (1 per 1,000 population) that usually has an onset between 45 and 65 years of age (1 per 100 in people > 65).
Management	**Levodopa** crosses the blood-brain barrier and is converted to dopamine in the CNS (side effects include dyskinesia, arrhythmias, nausea, vomiting, hypotension, and psychosis). It is usually administered with **carbidopa** (a dopamine decarboxylase inhibitor that does not cross the blood-brain barrier) to reduce the required dose of L-dopa and limit side effects. **Anticholinergics** are given

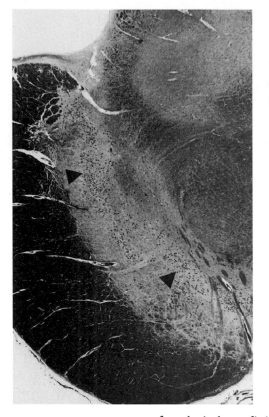 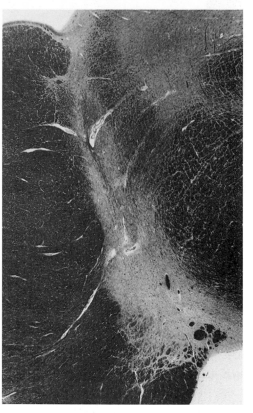

for their beneficial effect on rigidity and tremors (side effects include dry mouth, blurring of vision, urinary retention, and exacerbation of glaucoma); **amantadine** is used for mild disease, although its mechanism of action is not well understood (side effects include depression, anxiety, constipation, arrhythmias, and postural hypotension). **Bromocriptine** is a dopamine agonist associated with a lesser incidence of dyskinesia (side effects include digital vasospasm, nasal congestion, constipation, and worsening of peptic ulcer disease). **Selegiline** is a MAO-B inhibitor that prevents the breakdown of dopamine in the brain. **Surgery** includes implantation of adrenal medulla in the caudate nucleus, thalamotomy, or pallidotomy with variable results.

Complications Progressive disability and death.

Associated Diseases ◻ **Shy–Drager Syndrome** Autonomic system failure, possibly related to degeneration of presympathetic neurons; presents as orthostatic hypotension plus parkinsonism; treat with fludrocortisone, salt tablets and fluids to maintain intravascular volume; consider an alpha-agonist (e.g., pseudoephedrine).

ID/CC	A 65-year-old male who has been treated with **vincristine** for chronic lymphocytic leukemia complains of **tingling** (= PARESTHESIAS) of the hands and feet coupled with **constipation**.
HPI	The tingling began in his fingers two months ago with vincristine; only recently has he experienced tingling in the toes. The sensation is constant and does not change with movement or position.
PE	VS: normal. PE: speech appropriate; cranial nerves intact; motor strength 5/5; DTRs 2+ except 1+ in Achilles; Babinski's absent; **decreased pinprick sensation from midfoot and wrists distally;** proprioception and vibration intact.
Labs	ESR, B_{12}, folate, TSH, hemoglobin A_{1C}, and serum protein electrophoresis normal; reduction in sensory nerve action potential.
Imaging	N/A
Pathogenesis	Vinca alkaloids such as vincristine function as **mitotic spindle inhibitors** and interact with tubulin, resulting in the impairment of axonal transport.
Epidemiology	**Vincristine** is the chemotherapeutic agent that is most commonly associated with **peripheral neuropathy.** Other common causes of drug-induced peripheral neuropathies include **cisplatin** (pure sensory neuropathy), **taxol, dapsone** (pure motor, resembles amyotrophic lateral sclerosis), **ethionamide, INH, hydralazine, phenytoin,** and **adriamycin.**
Management	**Reduction or withdrawal** of vincristine should result in the remission of symptoms. If some residual paresthesia remains, symptomatic treatment can be initiated with **gabapentin** or **amitriptyline.** Stool softeners and mild cathartics may be given at the beginning of treatment.
Complications	If not properly identified and if vincristine is not discontinued, the neuropathy will progress. This will result in eventual axonal damage, causing **motor weakness.** The sensory neuropathy will also worsen, extending further up the arms and legs. Acute **intestinal ileus** and **bladder neuropathies** (serious autonomic

PERIPHERAL NEUROPATHY DUE TO VINCRISTINE

involvement) are two absolute contraindications to continued vincristine therapy.

Associated Diseases ◙ **Diabetic Peripheral Neuropathy** Insidious loss of peripheral or cranial nerve function related to chronic hyperglycemia; presents with numbness, tingling, and burning in the lower extremities in a stocking-glove distribution; EMG shows denervation; treat with insulin for strict glycemic control (monitor with hemoglobin A1c levels); add carbamazepine for pain; emphasize foot care to patients to prevent the development of ulcers.

◙ **Vitamin B12 deficiency** Cofactor for DNA and myelin synthesis; deficiency is due to malabsorption (sprue, enteritis, *Diphyllobothrium latum* infection), absence of intrinsic factor (pernicious anemia), prolonged dietary deficiency (as in vegans), or terminal ileum disease; presents with anemia, degenerative changes in the spinal cord (especially the posterior columns and the corticospinal tracts), and peripheral neuropathies; hypersegmented PMNs, megaloblastic RBCs, and decreased serum vitamin B_{12}; treat the underlying disorder, IM vitamin B_{12}.

PERIPHERAL NEUROPATHY DUE TO VINCRISTINE

ID/CC	A **65-year-old** female says that her family has noted a one-year history of **marked personality change** and **speech difficulty.**
HPI	The patient's family claims that she is no longer interested in her hobbies of golf and reading. She now becomes angry for no apparent reason.
PE	VS: normal. PE: impaired cognitive function; CN II–XII intact; motor strength 5/5, DTRs 2+; prominent snout and grasp reflex noted.
Labs	Serum B_{12}, folate, and TSH normal; VDRL negative.
Imaging	MR-Brain: marked **bilateral frontotemporal atrophy.**
Pathogenesis	Pathologic examination reveals **atrophy** of gray and white matter in the **frontal and temporal lobes.** The characteristic lesions are argentophilic **Pick bodies.**
Epidemiology	N/A
Management	No specific treatment. Typically progresses over 3–15 years.
Complications	With progression of disease, complications are primarily **infectious** and include aspiration pneumonia, UTIs, and decubitus ulcers.
Associated Diseases	N/A

ID/CC	An **18-year-old female** complains of **headache, vomiting,** and **blurred vision** for the past 2–3 weeks.
HPI	The patient experiences the headache as a "pressure-like" feeling in the parietal region bilaterally. She also experienced intermittent brief loss of vision while bending. She denies any associated photophobia or phonophobia.
PE	VS: normal. PE: **papilledema;** neck supple; neurologic exam otherwise normal.
Labs	CBC: normal. LP: **opening pressure elevated** (34 cm H_2O); no white cells; normal protein and glucose.
Imaging	CT-Head: no mass, hemorrhage, or midline shift; normal ventricle size (may even be small). MR-Venography: normal (rules out transverse and sagittal sinus thrombosis).
Pathogenesis	The condition is idiopathic; **overproduction of CSF and impairment of CSF absorption** by the arachnoid villi may be involved. Pseudotumor can follow corticosteroid withdrawal or excesses of vitamin A or tetracycline.
Epidemiology	Incidence is higher in **women** between the ages of 15 and 44.
Management	Withdrawal of precipitating agent. Treatment with **acetazolamide** causes decreased CSF production; if not tolerated, **furosemide** may be used. Serial LPs have a role if no medications can be tolerated. If visual loss continues despite medical therapy, then consider optic nerve sheath fenestration or **CSF shunting.**
Complications	**Optic atrophy** causing **permanent visual loss;** electrolyte abnormalities due to diuretic therapy.
Associated Diseases	◨ **Meningioma** The most common benign extra-axial CNS tumor in adults; presents with focal neurologic deficits, vision changes, headache, nausea, and vomiting; MR or CT demonstrates mass lesion; histology demonstrates whorled appearance and psammoma bodies; treat with surgical resection; excellent prognosis. ◨ **Normal Pressure Communicating Hydrocephalus** Idiopathic or secondary to compromised CSF absorption (meningitis, SAH); presents with dementia, gait ataxia,

and incontinence; CT/MR show enlarged lateral ventricles; treat with lumbar-peritoneal shunt.

◘ **Vitamin A Toxicity** Most often iatrogenic; presents with alopecia, skin scaling, orange discoloration, papilledema (pseudotumor cerebri), hyperkeratosis, and hepatomegaly; XR of long bones and spine shows subcortical hyperostosis; treat with moderation of vitamin A intake.

ID/CC	A **4-year-old girl** has been having **episodes of persistent staring** during which she does not answer questions and **looks distracted.**
HPI	One of the child's cousins has had similar episodes. During the episodes, the child rolls her eyes upward, rhythmically nods her head, and drops objects from her hand.
PE	VS: normal. PE: neurologic exam normal; under hyperventilation and strobe light, patient was shown to have fine, twitching movements of the eyelids, pupillary dilatation (= MYDRIASIS), tachycardia, and piloerection.
Labs	CBC: normal. SaO_2 98%. Lytes/LFTs/UA: normal. Calcium normal. [A] EEG: during seizure, **bursts of 3-cycle-per-second** spike-and-wave activity occur; in the interictal period, EEG is normal.
Imaging	CT-Head: no organic pathology.
Pathogenesis	Also called petit mal seizures, absence seizures are inherited as an **autosomal-recessive** trait and are characterized by an idiopathic, temporary (usually < 10-sec) **loss of awareness** that is **not preceded by an aura** and is followed by a characteristic abrupt regaining of consciousness. Hyperventilation and blinking strobe lights may precipitate the attacks.
Epidemiology	**Higher incidence in children** aged 3–13 years; more common among girls. Petit mal seizures never begin after age 20.
Management	Most patients show a **benign course,** with symptoms disappearing by puberty. **Ethosuximide** and **valproic acid** are useful drugs; a ketogenic or medium-chain triglyceride diet will also help.
Complications	Loss of capacity to speak and understand with a prolonged absence seizure (= PETIT MAL STATUS).
Associated Diseases	N/A

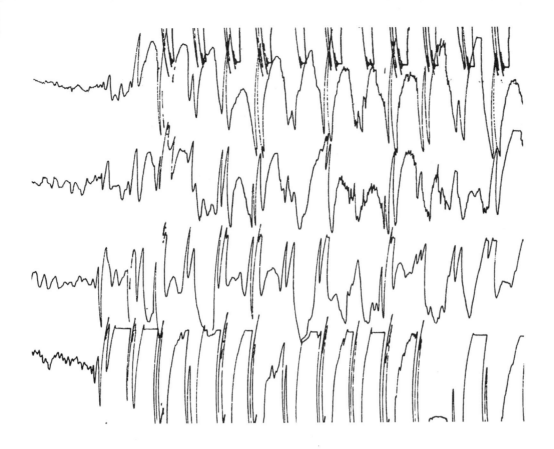

SEIZURE – ABSENCE

ID/CC	A 16-year-old **male** is brought to the physician by his mother, who reports two recent episodes during which she observed her son to be "out of it."
HPI	When he was a baby, the patient had **herpes encephalitis** (birth injuries, head trauma, childhood febrile convulsions, and CNS malignancies may cause seizures). He has required remedial reading and math classes since the third grade. His episodes began when he complained of an unpleasant smell **(aura)**, suddenly stopped talking, and **"stared straight ahead"**; his mouth was also twitching. Each episode was over in approximately two minutes, after which the patient was **confused and sleepy** (= POSTICTAL CONFUSION). After taking a nap, he returned to normal. There is no family history of seizures, and the patient denies any alcohol or drug use.
PE	VS: normal. PE: no focal neurologic deficits.
Labs	CBC: normal. SaO_2 99%. Lytes: normal. Toxicology screen negative. EEG: normal background with **focal spike discharges over left temporal lobe;** no frank seizure activity.
Imaging	MR-Brain: **left medial temporal sclerosis.**
Pathogenesis	Complex partial seizures are also referred to as **"temporal lobe"** or **"psychomotor"** epilepsy. Unlike simple partial seizures, they always involve loss of consciousness and frequently **follow auditory or olfactory auras.** Medial temporal sclerosis is a scar tissue that in this case resulted from the patient's childhood encephalitis; **scar tissue serves as a focus for seizure activity.** The cause of most seizure disorders is idiopathic, and seizures may occur unpredictably without any precipitating cause. However, external factors that may lower the seizure threshold include lack of sleep, missed meals, stress, alcohol or other drugs, fever, and specific stimuli such as flickering lights.
Epidemiology	Epilepsy shows a **male predominance** and is most common in the first decade of life and then after the age of 60.
Management	**Phenytoin** and **carbamazepine** are equally effective in treating complex partial seizures; the choice of drug is

based on its side effect profile. The primary side effects of phenytoin are gingival hyperplasia, ataxia, and hepatotoxicity; those of carbamazepine are leukopenia, nausea, and vomiting.

Complications

Secondary generalization of seizure that began as a complex partial seizure; serious injury during seizure episode; and **status epilepticus.**

Associated Diseases

N/A

ID/CC	A **10-month-old child** is rushed to the emergency room because of sudden loss of consciousness, rigidity of muscles followed by **jerky movements of all limbs, upward rolling of the eyes, and urination.**
HPI	The patient was being treated for **severe otitis media** with **high fever** and had a 40.2 C temperature when the seizure began.
PE	VS: **fever** (38.1 C). PE: neck supple; pupils equal, round, and reactive to light; no focal neurologic signs; severe otitis media in right ear.
Labs	CBC: leukocytosis with left shift. SaO_2 98%. Lytes/UA: normal. LP: CSF normal. EEG: posterior asymmetric slowing of background.
Imaging	CT-Brain: normal.
Pathogenesis	Febrile seizures are those that occur in children **< 5 years** and **> 3 months of age,** have **no organic cause,** and are precipitated by a high fever.
Epidemiology	There is usually a family history of the disease, and recurrence occurs in 30% of patients.
Management	**Temperature control with acetaminophen** and cold baths. **Diazepam** may be used in the acute setting to control seizures. Treat the precipitating illness with appropriate antibiotics.
Complications	**Recurrence** (occurs more often in those with a young age at onset, those with a family history, seizures with a lower temperature level, and children with marked slowing on EEG), mental deficiency, **developmental disturbances** (more so in patients with previous neurologic disturbance and with focal seizures), **status epilepticus,** and **epilepsy** development (rare).
Associated Diseases	N/A

ID/CC	A 16-year-old male presents with sudden **loss of consciousness** and muscle hypertonia followed by **rhythmic movements of the limbs** with upward rolling of the eyes, tongue biting, and urinary incontinence; he is now in a state of confusion and lethargy.
HPI	He is otherwise healthy and is a good student. He has two cousins who suffer from a seizure disorder. He does not take any illicit drugs or medications.
PE	VS: normal. PE: lethargic; complains of headache but is awake and oriented; no cyanosis; lesion on anterior third of tongue attributed to bite during seizure; nonfocal neurologic examination.
Labs	CBC/LFTs: normal. SaO$_2$ 99%. Lytes: normal. UA: tox screen negative. **Prolactin elevated** (it does not rise after a psychogenic tonic-clonic "seizure"). ECG: normal sinus rhythm. **[A]** EEG: diffuse slowing with generalized spike-and-wave pattern. LP: CSF normal.
Imaging	CT-Head: no apparent intracranial pathology.
Pathogenesis	Grand mal seizures are also called generalized tonic-clonic seizures. A tonic-clonic seizure can begin as a partial complex seizure, in which case it is termed partial complex seizure secondarily generalized.
Epidemiology	Half of patients who suffer a new-onset tonic-clonic seizure will have a recurrence. Epilepsy may remit spontaneously in up to one-third of cases and may be controlled with medications.
Management	Start with a low dose of **valproic acid** (side effects include severe, fatal hepatotoxicity, pancreatitis, thrombocytopenia, hair loss, GI upset, and tremors) and increase dosage slowly; the vast majority of cases can be controlled with a single drug. If not effective despite therapeutic blood levels, the addition of **phenytoin** (side effects include numerous drug interactions, gingival hyperplasia, allergy, leonine facies, ataxia, hirsutism, peripheral neuropathy, rash, megaloblastic anemia, lung fibrosis, and osteoporosis), **phenobarbital** (side effects include sedation, numerous drug interactions), **carbamazepine** (side effects include GI upset, thrombocytopenia, aplastic anemia, rash, nystagmus, and diplopia), or primidone (main side effect is sedation) may

be helpful. When the patient has been seizure-free on medications for two years, tapering may be attempted in the knowledge that recurrence is likely.

Complications **Chronicity,** difficulty controlling seizure activity, **status epilepticus** (single seizure lasting > 30 minutes or a series of seizures with no return to consciousness lasting > 30 minutes), and **motor vehicle accidents.**

Associated Diseases N/A

ID/CC	A 66-year-old male with **lung cancer** is discovered "**shaking**" in bed and unable to speak.
HPI	The patient was diagnosed with lung cancer six months ago and has been treated with chemotherapy. He has complained of severe early-morning **headaches** associated with **nausea and projectile vomiting,** which improve as the day progresses, coupled with **blurred vision** (due to papilledema). Now he is confused, but his right arm and leg are no longer shaking.
PE	VS: normal. PE: alert and oriented; able to follow commands; **4/5 strength in right** arm and leg with 5/5 strength on left; **bilateral papilledema.**
Labs	CBC: anemia. SaO_2 97%. Lytes: normal. Troponin I normal.
Imaging	[A] CT-Head (with contrast): **ring-enhancing lesion** (1) in the **left parietal region** with surrounding mild edema.
Pathogenesis	The metastatic lesion serves as the seizure focus. Symptoms are due to edema surrounding the mass and destruction of brain tissue by the metastases.
Epidemiology	Fifteen percent of patients with diagnosed cancer develop cerebral metastases (40% are single lesions). **Malignancies that metastasize to the brain** are **lung, breast, melanoma, renal cell,** and **colon.**
Management	Administer **lifelong antiepileptic treatment (phenytoin);** obtain an MR of the brain to determine the possible presence of one or more metastatic lesions. In the presence of a **single brain lesion** and if the patient is in relatively good health, **resection** will improve life span. If the patient is in poor health or has **multiple metastatic lesions** of the brain, then **radiation** (breast and small cell lung cancer metastases respond well; melanoma and kidney adenocarcinoma metastases are resistant to radiotherapy) and steroids (IV dexamethasone) should be used to reduce the edema surrounding the lesion.
Complications	Recurrent seizures after treatment due to persistence or further growth of tumor, severe headaches, altered mental status, and increasing neurologic deficits.
Associated Diseases	◘ **Neurocysticercosis** Results from ingesting eggs of

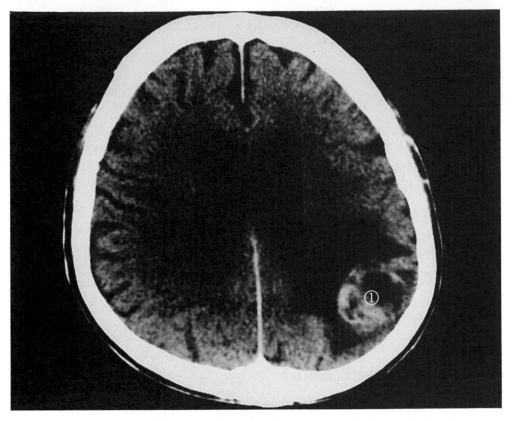

Taenia solium (pork tapeworm) through fecally contaminated food or autoinfection; associated with a history of travel to an endemic area (e.g., Latin America); presents with seizures and focal neurologic deficits; subcutaneous calcifications; CT/MR show intracranial cysts or calcifications; serology positive; treat with praziquantel or albendazole plus corticosteroids.

ID/CC	A **32-year-old male** fell two stories from the roof of a house and is now **unable to get up or move his legs.**
HPI	The patient was previously healthy.
PE	VS: normal. PE: able to follow commands; speech appropriate; cranial nerves intact; 5/5 strength in upper extremities; **0/5 motor strength in lower extremities;** DTRs 2+ in upper extremities; DTRs absent in lower extremities (may increase later); **no sensation to pinprick below iliac crest** (T12 sensory level); **rectal tone markedly diminished.**
Labs	N/A
Imaging	MR-Spine: fracture-dislocation of the T12 vertebral body with compression of the spinal cord (the majority of thoracolumbar fractures occur between T12 and L2).
Pathogenesis	There are **four types** of spinal injury: flexion, extension, axial due to compressive force, and rotational. Spinal cord injury can result in neurogenic shock, when the sympathetic innervation to the vasculature is compromised; patients experience hypotension and bradycardia.
Epidemiology	**Younger men** are at highest risk. Associated with a mortality rate of 5%–20%; quadriplegia is the end result in 30%–40% of cases.
Management	ABCs; **mechanical stabilization** of the entire spine to prevent further injury. Administer **IV methylprednisolone** within 24 hours of injury to minimize edema. **Surgery** should be conducted for permanent stabilization of the spine and baclofen given for muscle spasms. Intermittent straight catheterization due to urinary incontinence. Insertion of nasogastric tube.
Complications	Autonomic dysfunction, respiratory and skin infections due to immobility, urinary incontinence, UTIs, painful muscle spasms, and constipation requiring daily bowel regimen (stool softener, enemas).
Associated Diseases	N/A

....

42.   **SPINAL CORD INJURY DUE TO TRAUMA**

ID/CC	A **10-year-old** male presents with a **severe headache** that does not respond to analgesics, along with **projectile vomiting.**
HPI	In the ER, he suffered a **seizure.** The headache was present upon awakening. Directed questioning reveals that he has been behaving oddly for the past month.
PE	VS: normal. PE: appears confused; **ataxic gait; papilledema** and **nystagmus;** mild hypotonia of left arm; cardiopulmonary and abdominal exams normal.
Labs	CBC: normal. SaO_2 99%. Lytes: normal. UA: normal. LP/LFTs: normal. TFTs normal.
Imaging	**[A]** CT-Head: enhancing, irregular **cerebellar mass** (1) with cystic areas in the left posterior cranial fossa. **[B]** MR-Brain (sagittal): another posterior fossa enhancing astrocytoma.
Pathogenesis	Astrocytomas are **slow-growing** (with the exception of grade 4 astrocytoma, or glioblastoma multiforme), **malignant brain tumors** that **originate from neuroectodermal neuroglia;** in children they are usually **located in the cerebellum,** whereas in adults they are located in the cerebrum. Astrocytomas are commonly cystic in children, and their growth may cause increased ICP, seizures, and hydrocephalus.
Epidemiology	Brain tumors are the second most common cause of childhood cancer. Cerebellar astrocytomas are the **most common primary brain tumors in childhood** (followed by medulloblastoma and ependymoma). There is a higher incidence of astrocytomas in children with previous CNS irradiation, neurofibromatosis, and tuberous sclerosis as well as in children with a family history. Age < 4 years is an unfavorable prognostic sign.
Management	Stage the disease with CSF analysis, MRI, and angiography if necessary. **Dexamethasone** is used to decrease brain edema, and **phenytoin** is used as an anticonvulsant. **Surgical resection** depends on the location of the tumor. Most patients will eventually need radiation. Chemotherapy may temporarily control the disease, allowing radiotherapy to be postponed to a later age, when outcomes are better.
Complications	**Hydrocephalus, seizures,** herniation, functional loss,

ASTROCYTOMA

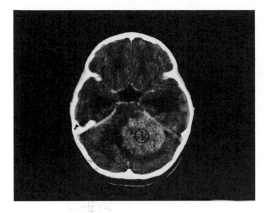
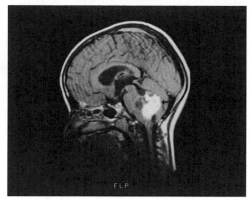

and irradiation damage (neuropsychological disturbances, hypothyroidism, growth retardation).

Associated Diseases

◻ **Glioblastoma** The most common primary brain tumor in adults; presents with acute-onset focal neurologic deficits, projectile vomiting, and headache; MR or CT reveals a large, irregular ring-enhancing mass lesion in the cerebral hemisphere; treat with radiation therapy or surgical excision for palliation only; recurrence and death are extremely common.

◻ **Medulloblastoma** The most common brain tumor in children; usually cerebellar; presents with subacute-onset headache, ataxia, projectile vomiting, and focal neurologic deficits; MR or CT reveals mass lesion; treat with radiation therapy; recurrence is common.

◻ **Oligodendroglioma** A slow-growing glial tumor; uncommon; presents with focal neurologic findings, nausea, vomiting, and headache; head CT shows a round, calcified, hypodense lesion; treat with surgery and radiotherapy.

ID/CC	A 16-year-old boy presents with **short stature** and **delayed onset of puberty.**
HPI	He also complains of **intolerance to cold, easy fatigability, dry skin,** and **constipation.** Directed questioning reveals that he has also been suffering from **polyuria.**
PE	VS: normal. PE: short for age; papilledema and optic disk swelling (due to increased ICP) as well as **bitemporal hemianopsia** (due to impingement on optic chiasm).
Labs	CBC: normal. Low T3, T4, and TSH. Lytes: hypernatremia. UA: low specific gravity (< 1.006) (due to diabetes insipidus).
Imaging	**[A]** CT-Head: small, calcified suprasellar mass. **[B]** CT-Head (contrast): large cystic craniopharyngioma. MR: classically, an enhancing **cystic, multilobulated suprasellar mass with ring calcification;** hydrocephalus (due to obstruction of foramen of Munro and aqueduct of Sylvius).
Pathogenesis	Craniopharyngioma is a tumor that is embryologically derived from squamous cell **remnants of Rathke's pouch.** It is usually located in the suprasellar region and **causes growth retardation, diabetes insipidus** (due to compression of the pituitary), **bitemporal hemianopsia** (due to pressure on the optic chiasm), and **headache** (due to obstructive hydrocephalus). The clinical significance of this histologically benign tumor lies in its proximity to the optic chiasm, the carotid arteries, CN III, and the pituitary stalk.
Epidemiology	The **most common supratentorial brain tumor in children;** has a bimodal age distribution with a second peak in incidence in the fifth decade of life.
Management	**Needle aspiration** has the lowest morbidity but is associated with a higher recurrence rate; **radiation** is always needed if aspiration is chosen. **Surgical resection** of as much tumor as possible without endangering the endocrine and intellectual functions with postoperative radiotherapy is the usual treatment. Hydrocortisone is usually given in the perioperative period.
Complications	Necrosis of the pituitary stalk during surgery with

CRANIOPHARYNGIOMA

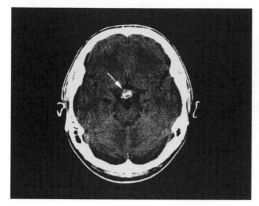 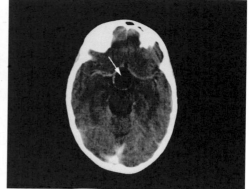

release of ADH and a sharp decrease in urinary volume; postoperative recurrence of tumor.

Associated Diseases   N/A

ID/CC	A **78-year-old** male nursing-home resident suffers a generalized seizure.
HPI	The patient has never had a seizure before. He has experienced **headaches** that are worse in the morning and admits to occasional **nausea and vomiting.**
PE	VS: **hypertension** (BP 150/90). PE: exhibits confusion postictally; neck supple; **bilateral papilledema; Babinski's present on right side;** normal lung and skin exam.
Labs	CBC normal.
Imaging	[A] CT-Head: single, irregular enhancing left temporoparietal mass lesion with necrotic center (1), mass effect (2), and moderate surrounding edema.
Pathogenesis	Glioblastoma multiforme is a **grade 4 astrocytoma** and is **markedly anaplastic.** Almost 75% of adult brain tumors are **supratentorial,** and the rest are in the posterior fossa. Histopathology reveals abundant necrosis.
Epidemiology	Occurs more commonly in **elderly individuals,** with a peak incidence in the seventh decade.
Management	**Tumor staging** is performed with CSF analysis, MRI, and angiography; **dexamethasone** is given to decrease brain edema; **phenytoin** is given as an anticonvulsant. Eventual surgical resection is planned depending on the location and extent of the tumor. Radiation and chemotherapy usually follow.
Complications	Hydrocephalus, seizures, herniation, and functional loss.
Associated Diseases	◘ **Meningioma** The most common benign extra-axial CNS tumor in adults; presents with focal neurologic deficits, vision changes, headache, nausea, and vomiting; MR or CT demonstrates mass lesion; histology demonstrates whorled appearance and psammoma bodies; treat with surgical resection; excellent prognosis.
	◘ **Metastatic Brain Tumors** Commonly caused by lung, breast, melanoma, kidney, and GI mets; presents with acute-onset focal neurologic deficits, headache, nausea, vomiting, and altered mental status; MR and CT show small, well-circumscribed lesions at white-gray

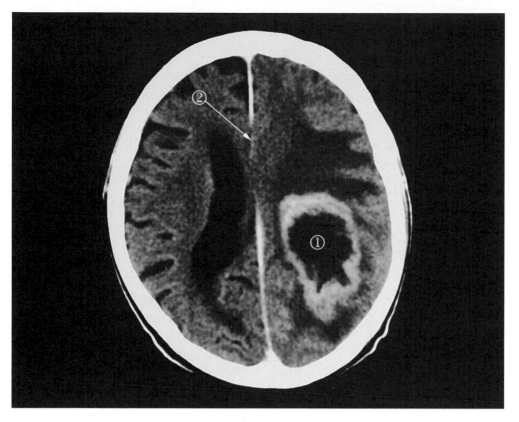

junction; treat with local irradiation; treat underlying malignancy.

◻ **Oligodendroglioma** A slow-growing glial tumor; uncommon; presents with focal neurologic findings, nausea, vomiting, and headache; head CT shows a round, calcified, hypodense lesion; treat with surgery and radiotherapy.

ID/CC	A 4-year-old boy presents with headache and awkward gait.
HPI	His symptoms have been present for three months. His parents have noted that he "walks into the wall." Over the past week, he has vomited daily.
PE	VS: normal. PE: bilateral papilledema; strength 5/5 throughout; ataxic gait; neck supple.
Labs	CBC/Lytes: normal. PT/PTT normal.
Imaging	[A] CT-Head: midline cerebellar mass (1) with surrounding edema and enlarged ventricles. [B] CT-Head (contrast): another case with an enhancing cerebellar vermis mass (1) and obstructive hydrocephalus.
Pathogenesis	Medulloblastoma arises from the floor of the fourth ventricle and may block the flow of CSF, resulting in increased ICP.
Epidemiology	Twenty-five percent of childhood brain tumors are medulloblastomas. The male-to-female ratio is 2 to 1; five-year survival is 50%.
Management	Surgery is performed to establish the diagnosis and debulk the tumor. Then radiotherapy is initiated. Adjuvant chemotherapy is experimental.
Complications	Radiotherapy may lead to cognitive delay as well as to endocrine abnormalities. Metastasis to meninges and spinal cord.
Associated Diseases	N/A

MEDULLOBLASTOMA

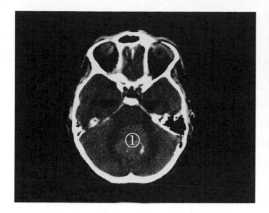 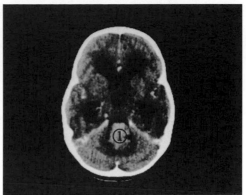

MEDULLOBLASTOMA

ID/CC	A **2-year-old girl** is brought to the ER by her parents, who have noticed a **bumpy right-sided abdominal mass.**
HPI	She is a healthy child who is up to date in her vaccinations. For the past week, her parents have noted the abdominal mass and occasional **diarrhea** (due to increased secretion of vasoactive intestinal peptide).
PE	VS: normal. PE: playful and in no acute distress; large right-sided abdominal mass with hard, irregular surface.
Labs	CBC: normal. UA: **elevated vanillylmandelic acid** (VMA is a catecholamine metabolite).
Imaging	MR-Brain: normal. MR-Spine: normal. CT-Abdomen: **solid mass within the right adrenal gland** that enhances with contrast. CT-Chest and Pelvis: normal. Nuc: normal.
Pathogenesis	Neuroblastoma **arises from primitive neural crest cells** that form the adrenal medulla and the cervical and thoracic sympathetic chains. Approximately 70% of neuroblastomas **produce norepinephrine and its metabolites; 75% originate in the retroperitoneal area** and 55% originate in the adrenal gland. Poor prognosis is associated with *N-myc* overexpression, which is associated with a deletion of the short arm of chromosome 1.
Epidemiology	A common childhood tumor. Mean age of onset is 20 months. Two-thirds of cases occur within the **first five years of life.**
Management	Management consists of intensive surveillance of the entire body for metastases (spinal cord, retroperitoneal sympathetic ganglia, posterior mediastinum), **surgical resection** of any solid tumor (adrenal gland, brain), **chemotherapy** (vincristine, cyclophosphamide), and **radiotherapy.**
Complications	Complications include invasion of abdominal organs and metastases to **liver, lung,** and **bone.** Immunosuppression from chemotherapy and radiotherapy may cause subsequent opportunistic infections.
Associated Diseases	◘ **Wilms' Tumor** Also called nephroblastoma; the most common abdominal malignancy in children; associated

with Beckwith–Wiedemann syndrome, hemihypertrophy, and sporadic aniridia; presents with a palpable abdominal mass and hypertension; diagnosis is via CT and US (evenly echogenic mass); requires surgical excision with local irradiation or chemotherapy for metastases.

ID/CC	A **26-year-old male** complains of having **"terrible headaches"** for the past five years.
HPI	The headaches usually occur at night and generally start with a burning in the right eye that, within minutes, involves the right orbit and right temple. The pain feels like a "hot poker" behind the right eye; the right eye then starts tearing and the right nostril begins to run. The pain lasts for 45 minutes. The patient generally has **3–4 attacks within a 24-hour period every six months.** He states that the **symptoms usually occur after** consumption of **alcohol.**
PE	VS: normal. PE: neurologic exam normal; during an acute episode, ptosis, miosis, anhidrosis, and enophthalmos of the right eye are present (= HORNER'S SYNDROME).
Labs	CBC: normal. ESR normal.
Imaging	MR/CT-Brain: no intracranial lesion or hemorrhage; no significant abnormality.
Pathogenesis	The pathology of cluster headache is thought to be vascular in nature. The neurotransmitter **substance P** may mediate the pain.
Epidemiology	Cluster headaches usually occur in **patients in their 20s** and is much more common in **males.** Many patients report that attacks **occur at the same time of year** (e.g., January and July).
Management	Prophylactic treatment consists of **verapamil** or **methysergide** for 1–2 months (methysergide should not be prescribed for longer periods owing to the risk of retroperitoneal fibrosis). Prednisone, ergotamine, and lithium are also used for prophylactic treatment. **Abortive therapy** consists of 100% **high-flow oxygen** at 8–10 L/min or **sumatriptan.**
Complications	Recurrence and persistence into late life.
Associated Diseases	◻ **Migraine** The second most common cause of headache in the U.S.; more common in women; precipitated by stress, sleeplessness, and anxiety; presents with recurring, usually unilateral headache with or without associated neurologic deficits, prodromal aura, visual flashing lights, nausea, and photosensitivity; treat

acutely with NSAIDs or sumatriptan; prophylaxis with beta-blockers, tricyclic antidepressants, or calcium channel blockers.

◩ **Tension Headache** A chronic disorder that is thought to result from contraction of the neck and scalp muscles; begins after age 20; presents with frequent bilateral, nonthrobbing headaches; treat with NSAIDs, relaxation techniques.

ID/CC	A **21-year-old female** presents with a history of **intermittent, severe headaches** of three years' duration.
HPI	The patient gets headaches approximately six times per year. The headaches begin with light flashes in the right visual field that last for 15–20 minutes; approximately 10 minutes later, a **unilateral** left **temporal throbbing pain** begins. The pain increases in severity and then lasts for 10–12 hours. Occasionally the headaches are **associated with nausea and vomiting.** In addition, the patient cannot bear light, movement, or noise. She has a **family history of migraine.**
PE	VS: stable. PE: funduscopy reveals sharp disks bilaterally; visual acuity 20/20 bilaterally; remainder of neurologic exam normal.
Labs	CBC/Lytes: normal. ESR normal (check for temporal arteritis).
Imaging	N/A
Pathogenesis	Individuals have noted various **precipitants** to migraines, including red wine, exercise, menstruation, estrogen, caffeine, lack of sleep, and skipping of meals. Migraine can occur with **aura** (a transient neurologic dysfunction, usually visual in nature, that occurs within 60 minutes before or after headache onset).
Epidemiology	Most commonly, the initial attack is during **teenage years.** More **common in females** after puberty.
Management	**Prophylaxis** with **beta-blockers, verapamil,** or **valproic acid. Abortive treatment** consists of **NSAIDs,** sumatriptan, and dihydroergotamine nasal spray.
Complications	N/A
Associated Diseases	◻ **Tension Headache** A chronic disorder that is thought to result from contraction of the neck and scalp muscles; begins after age 20; presents with frequent bilateral, nonthrobbing headaches; treat with NSAIDs, relaxation techniques.

ID/CC	A **70-year-old woman** presents with a **severe, intermittent right temporal headache** and **fever** of two months' duration and blurred vision in the right eye for two days.
HPI	The headache is neither relieved nor aggravated by changes in position or activity level. The patient also complains of **pain in the jaw when chewing** (= CLAUDICATION), weight loss, and discomfort on combing the right scalp but denies any associated nausea, vomiting, photophobia, or phonophobia. She has achieved some relief with acetaminophen.
PE	VS: mild fever; otherwise normal. PE: visual acuity normal; funduscopy reveals a swollen right disk; palpation reveals a right **temporal artery** that is **tender, pulseless, nodular,** and tortuous; locally tender scalp.
Labs	CBC: mild normocytic, normochromic anemia; mild leukocytosis and thrombocytosis. **Markedly elevated ESR** and acute phase reactants (C1-reactive protein); serum protein electrophoresis reveals mild polyclonal hypergammaglobulinemia; rheumatoid factor, ANA, and dsDNA negative (rules out connective tissue disorders); temporal artery biopsy positive; **biopsy reveals mononuclear cell infiltrates in the media,** particularly in the internal elastic lamina, as well as intimal thickening and granulomas containing multinucleated giant cells, histiocytes, and lymphocytes.
Imaging	N/A
Pathogenesis	The etiology is unknown. The histopathologic lesion is **giant-cell granuloma** within the vessel wall, leading to stenosis of the lumen. Involvement of an affected artery is patchy. Vascular inflammation is found most often in the superficial temporal arteries as well as in the vertebral, ophthalmic, and posterior ciliary arteries.
Epidemiology	Median age of onset is 75. More prevalent in females.
Management	**High-dose corticosteroids urgently** to prevent blindness; continue until symptoms resolve and ESR normalizes, and then taper slowly. Early temporal artery biopsy yields a definitive diagnosis. Most patients require a minimum of six months of therapy; some will require chronic steroid administration.

TEMPORAL ARTERITIS

Complications Complications include loss of vision and opportunistic infections (due to long-term prednisone treatment). Death may occur from strokes, ruptured aorta secondary to aortitis, and MI from coronary arteritis.

Associated Diseases ◘ **Optic Neuritis** Inflammation of the optic nerve, usually unilateral; associated with demyelinating diseases such as MS or viral etiologies; presents with orbital pain exacerbated by eye movement, unilateral vision loss, afferent pupillary defect, and scotomas; treat with corticosteroids.

ID/CC	A 62-year-old housewife complains of **recurrent episodes of headaches** that she has experienced since the age of 40.
HPI	Initially her headaches presented as a moderate squeezing pain in the **bilateral frontal area.** The headaches occurred twice monthly and were relieved with two acetaminophen tablets and a nap. For the past two years, the headaches have occurred 3–4 times a week, with accompanying nausea approximately 1–2 times a week. Minimal relief is obtained with ibuprofen. She denies associated phonophobia, photophobia, or focal motor deficits.
PE	VS: normal. PE: funduscopic exam reveals sharp disks bilaterally; visual acuity 20/20 bilaterally; neurologic exam normal.
Labs	ESR normal.
Imaging	CT-Head: no intracranial lesions or hemorrhage.
Pathogenesis	Overuse of OTC medications or depression may play a role. Chronic tension headache is characterized by pain that is **bilateral** in location and present for **> 15 days per month** for at least the last **six months;** it may or may not be accompanied by nausea, and there is no vomiting or photophobia. Pain is rarely throbbing in nature and is not aggravated by routine physical activity.
Epidemiology	N/A
Management	Add **amitriptyline** or gabapentin to NSAIDs or acetaminophen. Four to six weeks of treatment is necessary to determine efficacy.
Complications	Recurrent headaches.
Associated Diseases	◘ **Migraine** The second most common cause of headache in the U.S.; more common in women; precipitated by stress, sleeplessness, and anxiety; presents with recurring, usually unilateral headache with or without associated neurologic deficits, prodromal aura, visual flashing lights, nausea, and photosensitivity; treat acutely with NSAIDs or sumatriptan; prophylaxis with beta-blockers, tricyclic antidepressants, or calcium channel blockers.

....

51.   **TENSION HEADACHE**

■ **Cluster Headache** Men are affected more than women; mean age at onset is 25 years; presents with unilateral pain around the orbit, associated ipsilateral tearing, conjunctival injection, Horner's syndrome, and nasal stuffiness; attacks come in repeated groups over several days separated by weeks to months without recurrence; treat acutely with oxygen and NSAIDs, prophylaxis with beta-blockers or ergot alkaloids.

ID/CC	A **47-year-old** male complains of episodes of severe **pain in the right cheek** over the past year.
HPI	The pain is **electric in character** and **occurs while he is shaving.** Each episode lasts 2–4 minutes. At first, the episodes occurred daily for 3–4 days and then disappeared for two months. For the past three weeks, the pain has occurred every day.
PE	VS: normal. PE: mild touch in **right V2** (maxillary subdivision of trigeminal) **distribution** reproduces the painful episode; remainder of neurologic exam normal.
Labs	ESR normal.
Imaging	MR-Brain: normal.
Pathogenesis	Usually **idiopathic,** but may be caused by a meningioma that compresses the gasserian ganglion, by a schwannoma of the nerve, or by malignant infiltration of the skull base. V2 or V3 distributions are more commonly affected than V1. The typical course is relapsing/remitting over several years.
Epidemiology	Ninety percent of patients are **> 40 years old.**
Management	**Carbamazepine,** gabapentin, **phenytoin,** or baclofen. If the patient fails medical treatment, then multiple **surgical treatments** are available, including alcohol block of the branch of the trigeminal nerve that is painful as well as percutaneous thermocoagulation of the trigeminal nerve sensory root (the procedure of choice in the elderly).
Complications	N/A
Associated Diseases	N/A

TRIGEMINAL NEURALGIA

From the authors of *Underground Clinical Vignettes*

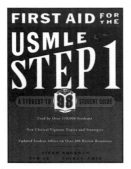

A true classic used by over 200,000 students around the world. The '99 edition features details on the new computerized test, new color plates and thoroughly updated high-yield facts and book reviews. Bi-directional links with the *Underground Clinical Vignettes Step 1* series. ISBN 0-8385-2612-8.

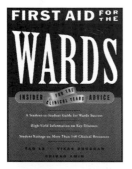

This high-yield student-to-student guide is designed to help students make the transition from the basic sciences to the hospital wards and succeed on their clinical rotations. The book features an orientation to the hospital environment, tips on being an effective and efficient junior medical student, student-proven advice tailored to each core rotation, a database of high-yield clinical facts, and recommendations for clinical pocket books, texts, and references. ISBN 0-8385-2595-4.

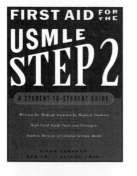

This entirely rewritten second edition now follows in the footsteps of *First Aid for the USMLE Step 1*. Features an exam preparation guide geared to the new computerized test, basic science and clinical high-yield facts, color plates and ratings of USMLE Step 2 books and software. Bi-directional links with the *Underground Clinical Vignettes Step 2* series.

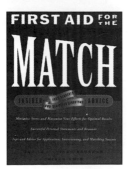

This top rated (5 stars, *Doody Review*) student-to-student guide helps medical students effectively and efficiently navigate the residency application process, helping them make the most of their limited time, money, and energy. The book draws on the advice and experiences of successful student applicants as well as residency directors. Also featured are application and interview tips tailored to each specialty, successful personal statements and CVs with analyses, current trends, and common interview questions with suggested strategies for responding. ISBN 0-8385-2596-2.

The *First Aid* series by Appleton & Lange...the review book leader.
Available through your local health sciences bookstore !